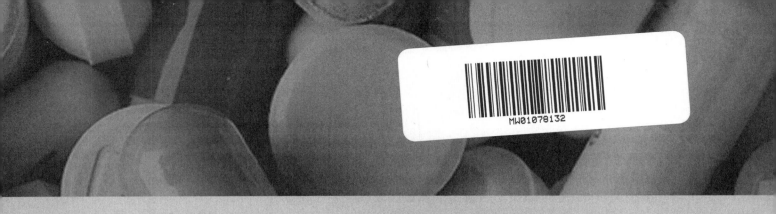

Workbook
for the
Manual for Pharmacy Technicians

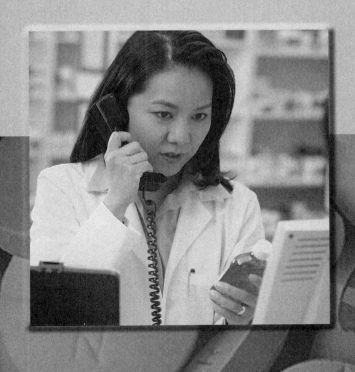

Mary McHugh

American Society of Health-System Pharmacists®

Any correspondence regarding this publication should be sent to the publisher, American Society of Health-System Pharmacists, 7272 Wisconsin Avenue, Bethesda, MD 20814, attention: Special Publishing.

The information presented herein reflects the opinions of the contributors and advisors. It should not be interpreted as an official policy of ASHP or as an endorsement of any product.

Because of ongoing research and improvements in technology, the information and its applications contained in this text are constantly evolving and are subject to the professional judgment and interpretation of the practitioner due to the uniqueness of a clinical situation. The editors, contributors, and ASHP have made reasonable efforts to ensure the accuracy and appropriateness of the information presented in this document. However, any user of this information is advised that the editors, contributors, advisors, and ASHP are not responsible for the continued currency of the information, for any errors or omissions, and/or for any consequences arising from the use of the information in the document in any and all practice settings. Any reader of this document is cautioned that ASHP makes no representation, guarantee, or warranty, express or implied, as to the accuracy and appropriateness of the information contained in this document and specifically disclaims any liability to any party for the accuracy and/or completeness of the material or for any damages arising out of the use or non-use of any of the information contained in this document.

Director, Special Publishing: Jack Bruggeman
Acquisitions Editor: Rebecca Olson
Senior Editorial Project Manager: Dana Battaglia
Production Editor: Johnna Hershey
Composition: Yvonne Yirka
Cover and Page Design: Carol Barrer

ISBN: 978-1-58528-257-9

Contents

Preface   v

Part One: Introduction to Pharmacy Practice   1

1. Introduction to Pharmacy   1
2. Pharmacy Law   7
3. Community and Ambulatory Care Pharmacy Practice   13
4. Hospital Pharmacy Practice   19
5. Home Care Pharmacy Practice   25
6. Specialty Pharmacy Practice   31
7. Drug Information Resources   35

Part Two: Foundation Knowledge and Skills   41

8. Communication and Teamwork   41
9. The Human Body: Structure and Function   47
10. Drug Classifications and Pharmacologic Actions   55
11. Basic Biopharmaceutics, Pharmacokinetics, and Pharmacodynamics   63
12. Medication Dosage Forms and Routes of Administration   69

Part Three: Practice Basics   75

13. Processing Medication Orders and Prescriptions   75
14. Pharmacy Calculations   79
15. Nonsterile Compounding and Repackaging   85
16. Aseptic Technique, Sterile Compounding, and IV Admixture Programs   91
17. Medication Errors   97

Part Four: Business Applications   103

18. Durable and Nondurable Medical Equipment, Devices, and Supplies   103
19. Purchasing and Inventory Control   109
20. Billing and Reimbursement   115

Answer Key   121

Index   195

Preface

New! Workbook for the Manual for Pharmacy Technicians

I have had the distinct honor of authoring the *Workbook for the Manual for Pharmacy Technicians*. Having worked in various pharmacist roles in both hospital and retail practice, I deeply respect the value of technicians. I have watched their roles expanding as the practice of pharmacy continually moves in new clinical directions. As a technician educator in an ASHP-accredited program, I value the authentic concepts and the organization of *The Manual for Pharmacy Technicians*. It is a great resource for training technicians.

In the *Workbook for the Manual for Pharmacy Technicians*, I have designed exercises to help students master the concepts and skills discussed in the *Manual*. By asking students to apply their knowledge, the exercises in the *Workbook* reinforce key points and allow for targeted assessment. Chapters in the *Workbook* complement those in the *Manual*, so that instructors and students can easily work between both books. Each chapter includes a wide range of exercises such as multiple choice, true/false, fill in the blank, concept and key term matching, short answer, and activity questions. I recommend using this book alongside the *Manual* to enhance learning.

Once you have learned the basics with the help of the *Manual* and the *Workbook*, the *Pharmacy Technician Certification Review and Practice Exam*, packaged with *TechPrep* cd, is helpful for those studying for certification.

I hope you find this *Workbook* a valuable resource for pharmacy technicians and educators.

Mary McHugh, PharmD

Chapter 1

Introduction to Pharmacy

Learning Outcomes

This chapter reinforces the following learning outcomes discussed in Chapter 1/ Introduction to Pharmacy of the *Manual for Pharmacy Technicians, 4th edition.*

- Compare and contrast the responsibilities of pharmacy technicians and pharmacists.
- Outline the differences among licensing, certification, and registration.
- Describe the advantages of formal training for pharmacy technicians.
- Describe the differences between the ambulatory and institutional pharmacy practice settings.
- List two specific examples each of ambulatory and institutional pharmacy practice settings.
- Describe at least six characteristics of a professional.
- List five tasks that pharmacy technicians perform in various pharmacy settings.
- Describe the concept of pharmaceutical care.
- Define medication therapy management.
- Explain why the use of outpatient pharmacy and medical services is increasing.

Multiple Choice 2

Matching 3

True or False 3

Fill in the Blank 4

Short Answer 4

Internet Research 4

Crossword Puzzle 5

Word Search 6

Multiple Choice

1. A pharmacy technician may perform all of the following tasks except:

   a. Refilling Pyxis.
   b. Repackaging medications.
   c. Maintaining medication inventory.
   d. Advising patients about aspirin.

2. Upon passing the exam provided by PTCB, pharmacy technicians earn a:

   a. Pharmacy Technician license.
   b. Pharmacy Technician registration.
   c. Pharmacy Technician diploma.
   d. Pharmacy Technician certificate.

3. Advantages of accredited pharmacy technician education include all of the following except:

   a. Provision of a separate credential to be used after the technician's name.
   b. Provision of standard educational goals designed to upgrade pharmacy technician education.
   c. Provision of basic competency of pharmacy technicians who graduate from an accredited program.
   d. Provision of criteria for technician trainees as they choose a technician training program.

4. Pharmacy technicians have the most patient contact in:

   a. Long-term care pharmacy.
   b. Hospital pharmacy.
   c. Nuclear pharmacy.
   d. Ambulatory pharmacy.

5. PBM stands for:

   a. Patient benefit manager.
   b. Pharmacy benefit manager.
   c. Patient behavior modification.
   d. Potential business model.

6. Medication therapy management (MTM) includes all of the following except:

   a. Assessment of a pharmacy's inventory.
   b. Formulation of a medication treatment plan.
   c. Selection, initiation, modification, or administration of medication therapy.
   d. Monitoring of a patient's response to therapy.

7. Pharmaceutical care includes all of the following except:

   a. Identification of potential and actual drug-related problems.
   b. Compounding sterile medications using aseptic techniques.
   c. Resolution of actual drug-related problems.
   d. Prevention of potential drug-related problems.

8. Pharmacokinetics is the study of:

   a. Drugs and their actions in the body.
   b. The process by which drugs are absorbed, distributed, metabolized, and eliminated in the body.
   c. The science of preparing and dispensing drugs.
   d. The movement of a prescription through the filling process.

9. In all states, pharmacists are licensed by the:

   a. NAPLEX.
   b. State Board of Pharmacy.
   c. NABP.
   d. PTCB.

10. ASHP's ten characteristics of a professional include all of the following except:

    a. Knowledge and skills of the profession.
    b. Commitment to self-improvement of skills and knowledge.
    c. Accountability for his or her work.
    d. Ability to defend medication errors.

11. Technician duties in a home care setting may include all of the following except:

    a. Preparing sterile injectable products.
    b. Maintaining computerized patient profiles.
    c. Delivering medications.
    d. Discussing drug interactions.

12. As the demand for cost-effective health care increases, pharmacy technicians with well-developed critical thinking skills may find themselves assuming responsibilities previously assigned to pharmacists such as:

    a. Managerial duties.
    b. Patient education.
    c. Pharmacokinetic studies.
    d. Drug utilization review.

Matching

A. Licensure

B. Registration

C. Certification

D. Accreditation

E. Hospital Pharmacy

F. Retail Pharmacy

G. MTM

H. ASHP

I. PTCB

J. AAPT

_____ 1. A nongovernmental agency or association grants recognition to an individual who has met certain predetermined qualifications specified by that agency or association. This recognition demonstrates to the public that the individual has achieved a certain level of knowledge, skill, or experience.

_____ 2. Granting recognition or vouching for conformance with established criteria (usually refers to recognition of an institution).

_____ 3. An agency of government grants permission to an individual to engage in a given occupation upon finding that the applicant has attained the minimal degree of competency necessary to ensure that the public health, safety, and welfare will be reasonably well protected.

_B_ 4. The process of making a list or being enrolled in an existing list.

_____ 5. Ambulatory pharmacy.

_____ 6. The organization that accredits Pharmacy Technician Training Programs.

_____ 7. A pharmacy technician organization.

_____ 8. A distinct service or group of services that optimize therapeutic outcomes for individual patients.

_____ 9. Institutional pharmacy.

_____ 10. An organization that provides a National Certification Test.

True or False

_____ 1. The study of how drugs are absorbed, distributed, metabolized, and eliminated by the body is called pharmacokinetics.

_____ 2. Educating patients about their medications or suggesting medication alternatives to physicians is a task for a pharmacy technician.

_____ 3. Training prerequisites for pharmacy technicians are the same throughout all of the states.

_____ 4. Only pharmacists may prepare and compound sterile products.

_____ 5. Technicians may be trained on the job or by completing a formal program.

_____ 6. Pharmacists may be trained on the job or by completing a formal program.

_____ 7. Pharmacy technicians must recertify every 2 years by completing 20 hours of continuing education, with at least 1 hour related to pharmacy law.

_____ 8. Pharmacy technician training programs are accredited by PTCB.

_____ 9. Residencies provide the opportunity for pharmacy technicians to gain clinical experience, usually in hospital, ambulatory, or community settings.

_____ 10. Most consumers believe that all pharmacy technicians have been trained and certified before they are allowed to prepare prescriptions.

_____ 11. There are three recognized certification tests—PTCE, ExCPT, and NPTE.

Fill in the Blank

1. To maintain certification, a pharmacy technician must accumulate _____ continuing education credits.

2. Pharmacy technicians must recertify every _____ years.

3. Of the required hours of continuing education, at least _____ hour(s) must be related to pharmacy law.

4. The PTCB exam has _____ questions.

5. The ExCPT exam has _____ questions.

6. A maximum of _____ hours may be earned at the technician's workplace under the direct supervision of a pharmacist.

7. _____ care is care that is given to those patients with incurable diseases who are generally not expected to live more than 6 months.

8. An example of institutional pharmacy is _____.

9. An example of ambulatory pharmacy is _____.

10. A _____ oversees prescription medication programs and processes and pays prescription medication insurance claims.

Short Answer

1. A customer comes into the pharmacy and needs some help finding OTC cough syrup. It is time for the technician's lunch break, and no one else is available. The technician tells the customer that the store is out of cough syrup so that he can go to lunch on time. Discuss the violations of professional conduct displayed by this pharmacy technician.

2. Discuss the typical pharmacy technician duties in different pharmacy settings such as community pharmacy and hospital pharmacy. What tasks might be the same and what tasks are unique in these settings?

3. What is the purpose of MTM (Medication Therapy Management) and how is it accomplished?

4. Compare and contrast the two organizations that offer a National Certification Exam for pharmacy technicians.

5. What is the organization that accredits Pharmacy Technician Training Programs?

6. Technicians may specialize in many areas. Describe the different specialty areas. Why would you be interested or not interested in these areas?

Internet Research

1. Go to www.PTCB.org and find out about the exam.

   a. How do you prepare for the exam?
   b. What is the content of the exam?
   c. How many questions are there?
   d. How long will you have for the test?

2. Go to the American Society of Health-System Pharmacists' web site, the pharmacy technician page at www.ashp.org/technicians.

   a. What are the opportunities for involvement in ASHP?
   b. What are ASHP's latest initiatives and activities?

3. Go to the National Association of Boards of Pharmacy web site at www.nabp.net.

   a. Find your State Board of Pharmacy Newsletter—what is new?
   b. Type "technician" in search box—what is new with technicians on the NABP web site?
   c. Click on "Government Affairs" and report any news about pharmacy technicians.

Crossword Puzzle

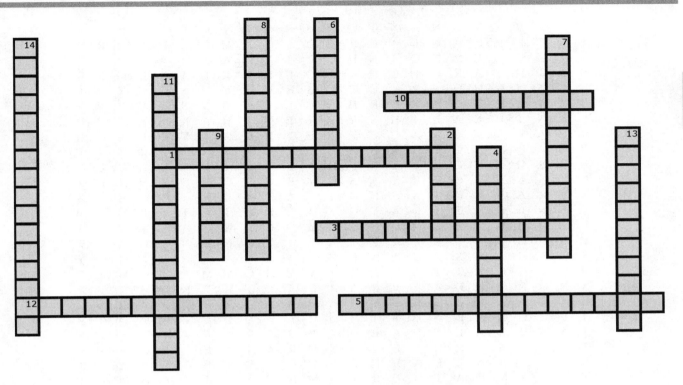

Across:

1. Technicians to check the work of other technicians
3. Granting recognition or vouching for
5. Nonsterile compounding
10. Provided by agency of the government
12. Critical skill in ambulatory pharmacy

Down:

2. Pharmacist degree
4. Dispensing cabinet
6. Pharmacist postgraduate training
7. The study of drugs
8. PTCB provides
9. Used in bar-code technology
11. Method of preparing sterile products
13. IV stands for
14. Study of movement of drug through body

Word Search

```
G I D N A R A N H N T C U H O S P I C E C E R E H
E N L E R R A C L A C I T U E C A M R A H P L R A
R A C C M E M C C I N H C E T Y C A M R A H P U A
H N T M T A R H E C H C A C E A R E E I C E M S R
N M T N C H O S P I C E C A R H I Y T N C M T N E
Y A T E P I C A C N R H A L L I C E N S U E L E N
E I N I H E A L T H S Y S T E M P H A R M A I C H
R H A P S M S A A C S F A E E N C A I T O E T C H
P H A R M A C Y B E N E F I T M A N A G E R Y I E
H A S O E A G T P T R E R A C E C I P S O H C L N
N I S L N T O E H Y A A C M R E T G N O L H R E R
R R R A A P C T A C N O I T A T I D E R C C A A S
P E S E C H C I R A Y C A I E R G I L T T S M N M
E M A H G T A E M M G L L R O N N N H A A Y I G I
F E E G A I H R A R S T A F I C C N H N C O A A E
S O A U A H S S C A A L O L I A H A A A T E A D Y
H G H I C E T T A H A R I Y M H C M M A I C U I E
I N C R E A H A A P R A A R I L T R T R O H R T E
H I T E A H O T E T T H A H A I A I R I P A L A U
I L C G N A R A M N I H G C F H D E L E R M D R P
I A T I D H E T E A P O I E P E R A I L Y N E T E
T I I S S N R D E L A T N M R A I E E L E R P S Y
A T A T T A E P A L U E E C C T L Y L C U P A I R
T N A R M R A T N E B T A M N T S Y I S A H M G T
I E E A C M I A C Y S E R E L R R I N N P R N E R
D D R T S P H A C Y I E D N O I Y E C I A M C R A
E E A I S A M A S O T E R E S E C M T A P P A A T
R R S O Y R M H A G R E T O I I A C C E M E M E I
C C H N A R T E N C P R T L L E O E E I R E R G
C H N H A L I O H O M E H E A L T H C A R E A A M
A A P H A H L O G E A E T M A L F T S A E P E H T
P H P E A A H O S P I T A L H A R M A C Y C Y O P
E R H E C A E R A C L A C I T U E C A M R A H P C
P H A R M E C I S T H E A H S G A Y H A C H E N L
C N H H O S P I T A L P H A R M A C Y M A I E O I
R T N S O E M T I H E O T I E M H H A R G R Y I E
```

ACCREDITATION
CREDENTIALING
HEALTHSYSTEMPHARMACY
HOMEHEALTHCARE
HOSPICECARE
HOSPITALPHARMACY
LICENSURE

LONGTERMCARE
PHARMACEUTICALCARE
PHARMACIST
PHARMACYBENEFITMANAGER
PHARMACYTECHNICIAN
REGISTRATION

Chapter 2

Pharmacy Law

Learning Outcomes

This chapter reinforces the following learning outcomes discussed in Chapter 2/ Pharmacy Law of the *Manual for Pharmacy Technicians, 4th edition.*

- Understand how the practice of pharmacy is regulated by federal and state laws and regulations and the role of State Boards of Pharmacy.
- Discuss state pharmacy laws and regulations that govern pharmacy technicians, including permitted functions and the requirements for pharmacy technician registration or licensure.
- Discuss the laws that regulate controlled substances, special requirements for pharmacy ordering and dispensing controlled substances, and the role of state prescription monitoring programs.
- Describe the restrictions on the sales of products containing pseudoephedrine and ephedrine.
- Describe the FDA approval process for drugs and the differences between brand name and generic drugs.
- Discuss generic drug substitution and the means for prescribers to indicate if substitution is not authorized.
- Discuss the difference between prescription drug inserts for prescribers and for patients.
- Discuss patient privacy in the pharmacy and the federal law that governs privacy of protected health information.

Multiple Choice 8

Matching 9

True or False 10

Fill in the Blank 10

Short Answer 11

Alphabet Soup 11

Word Search 12

Multiple Choice

1. The federal agency that administers and enforces federal laws for controlled substances and illegal substances such as narcotics and other dangerous drugs is the:

   a. FDA.
   b. DEA.
   c. NDA.
   d. NABP.

2. Biennial inventory is inventory of all controlled substances on hand to be conducted:

   a. Twice a year.
   b. Every 2 years.
   c. Once a year.
   d. Every 5 years.

3. Prescription monitoring programs are programs that collect, review, and analyze:

   a. Information received from pharmacies about controlled substance prescriptions dispensed in the state.
   b. Information from physicians about controlled substances prescribed in the state.
   c. Information from wholesalers about controlled substances purchased in the state.
   d. Information from insurance companies about controlled substance prescriptions dispensed in the state.

4. If state and federal laws or regulations differ:

   a. The state law has precedence.
   b. The federal law has precedence.
   c. The less strict of the two laws must be followed.
   d. Both laws must be followed, including the more stringent requirements.

5. Adhering to ethical principles means:

   a. "Doing the right thing."
   b. Complying with laws and regulations.
   c. Maintaining competency.
   d. Respecting patient privacy and confidentiality.
   e. All of the above.

6. State pharmacy laws are:

   a. Enacted by state legislatures through the legislative process.
   b. The same as rules and regulations.
   c. Issued and adopted by the NABP.
   d. All of the above.

7. The State Boards of Pharmacy have regulatory authority over a number of areas, including:

   a. Licensing pharmacies and pharmacists.
   b. Registering or licensing pharmacy technicians.
   c. Disciplinary actions against pharmacies, pharmacists, and pharmacy technicians for violations of pharmacy laws and regulations.
   d. All of the above.

8. Pharmacy technicians may:

   a. Provide patient counseling under the supervision of a pharmacist.
   b. Provide counseling if they are fluent in the patient's language.
   c. Are not authorized to counsel.
   d. Provide patient counseling under the supervision of a pharmacy intern.

9. Federal law allows Schedule III and IV prescriptions to be refilled:

   a. Up to 6 times within 5 months.
   b. Up to 5 times within 6 months.
   c. One time within 72 hours.
   d. Not refillable—require a new prescription for each filling.

10. Schedule V prescriptions may be refilled:

   a. As needed within 6 months.
   b. Five times within 6 months.
   c. One time within 72 hours.
   d. Not refillable—require a new prescription for each filling.
   e. None of the above.

Matching

A. Drug Price Competition and Patent Term Restoration Act (Hatch-Waxman Act)

B. Durham-Humphrey Amendment

C. FDA

D. Federal Food, Drug, and Cosmetic (FDC) Act of 1938

E. Food and Drug Act

F. Food and Drug Administration Modernization Act

G. Kefauver-Harris Drug Amendments

H. Medicare Prescription Drug Improvement and Modernization Act of 2003

I. Over-the-Counter Drug Review

J. Prescription Drug Marketing Act

K. Sherley Amendment

L. Tamper-resistant Packaging Regulations Licensure

_____ 1. Outlaws states from buying and selling food, drinks, and drugs that have been mislabeled and tainted.

_____ 2. Outlaws labeling drugs with fake medical claims meant to trick the buyer.

_____ 3. Food and Drug Administration.

_____ 4. Requires new drugs to be proven safe prior to marketing; starts a new system of drug regulation; requires safe limits for unavoidable poisonous substances; and allows for factory inspections.

_____ 5. Defines the type of drugs that cannot be used safely without medical supervision and limits the sale to prescription only by medical professionals.

_____ 6. Requires manufacturers to prove that their drugs are effective prior to marketing.

_____ 7. Non-prescription medications must be safe, effective, and appropriately labeled.

_____ 8. Makes it a crime to tamper with packaged products and requires tamper-proof packaging.

_____ 9. Allowed FDA to approve generic versions of brand-name drugs without repeating research to prove safety and efficacy; allowed brand-name drugs to apply for up to 5 years' additional patent protection for new drugs to make up for time lost while their products were going through the FDA approval process.

_____ 10. Designed to eliminate diversion of products from legitimate channels of distribution and requires wholesalers to be licensed.

_____ 11. Expands scope of agency activities and moves agency to the Department of Health and Human Services (DHHS).

_____ 12. Includes Medicare Part D, which increases access to medications through private insurers.

True or False

———— 1. DEA-registered pharmacies are required by law to take an initial inventory of all controlled substances on hand upon commencing operations or upon changes in ownership, with subsequent inventories conducted twice per year thereafter.

———— 2. The FDA is the federal agency that administers and enforces federal laws for controlled substances and illegal substances such as narcotics and other dangerous drugs.

———— 3. If state and federal laws or regulations differ, the state law has precedence.

———— 4. Pharmacy laws are enacted through the state legislature, and pharmacy rules and regulations are adopted through the State Board of Pharmacy.

———— 5. Pharmacy technician ratios refer to the numbers of training hours required for specialty practice.

———— 6. Patient counseling must be provided by the pharmacist.

———— 7. The federal law regulating controlled substances is the Federal Food, Drug, and Cosmetic (FDC) Act of 1938.

———— 8. An example of a Schedule II (CII) medication (one with high potential for abuse or misuse, high risk of dependence) is methylphenidate (Ritalin).

———— 9. The statement, "Caution: Federal law prohibits the transfer of this drug to any person other than the patient for whom it was prescribed," must be placed on all labels of legend drugs.

———— 10. Prescription monitoring programs monitor prescribing and dispensing of controlled substances.

———— 11. Ephedrine and pseudoephedrine, which are the active ingredients in common cough, cold, and allergy products, are precursor chemicals to cocaine and morphine.

———— 12. The primary federal law establishing health information privacy is the Health Insurance Portability and Accountability Act (HIPAA).

———— 13. Prescription monitoring programs have been implemented in all states.

Fill in the Blank

1. For a physician, the DEA number starts with either the letter _____ or the letter _____ followed by the first letter of the physician's last name.

2. The form used for ordering Schedule II controlled substances is called the DEA Form _____.

3. An example of a controlled substance that may be dispensed by a pharmacist in some states is a Schedule _____ cough syrup containing a limited amount of codeine.

4. If indicated by the prescriber, the maximum refills on a Schedule III prescription are _____ refills within _____ months after the date that the prescription was issued by the prescriber.

5. Federal law requires the pharmacy to keep controlled substance records for _____ years.

6. Federal law limits sales of pseudoephedrine products to _____ grams of these products in a 30-day period.

7. The regulating body, _____, approves all drugs that are available for distribution in the United States to assure that they are safe and effective.

8. When a generic drug delivers the same amount of the drug to the body in the same amount of time as the brand-name drug, it is said to be _____ to the brand-name drug.

9. The FDA's publication of therapeutically equivalent generic drugs, "Approved Drug Products with Therapeutic Equivalence Evaluations," is commonly called the _____.

10. Prescription drugs are also called "legend drugs" due to the federal law called _____ that mandated certain drugs to require a prescription and be labeled with the statement, "Caution: Federal law prohibits dispensing without a prescription."

11. Prescription drug products must include a _____ _____ that provides physicians, pharmacists, and other health care professionals with medical and scientific information about the prescription drug.

12. The child-resistant packaging test for hazardous products such as prescription drugs must demonstrate that _____ % of children cannot open the containers and that _____% of adults are able to open the containers without difficulty.

Short Answer

1. Your elderly customer, Mrs. Jones, brings her prescription to the pharmacy where you work. The prescription is written for Percocet 5/325. The physician has written 2 refills on the prescription, and Mrs. Jones has asked if she can have all refills filled today since she can't drive anymore and therefore it is very difficult to get to the pharmacy. What are the problems in this scenario and how should you respond?

2. A customer, Tom Smith, calls your pharmacy for a refill of his Lomotil prescription, which was originally filled January 5 of this year. The prescription was written for 30 tablets plus 8 refills. He has refilled his prescription every other month since the original filling in January. It is now July 5 of the same year. Explain what you would do and why.

3. A physician wants to call in a C-II prescription for MSContin for his patient. He says he will mail in a signed prescription the next day. Under what circumstances would this be okay?

4. Gail Gibson travels to other cities frequently and originally had her Lortab prescription filled at your pharmacy. It was transferred to a pharmacy in another city last month. Now that she is back in town, she would like this prescription transferred back to your pharmacy. What should you do?

5. Discuss the purpose of counseling patients. What types of information should pharmacists include when counseling patients?

6. List two OTCs (over-the-counter medications) that can be used in the manufacture of methamphetamine.

7. OTC medication labels should include specific information for the patient. Find an OTC medication in your home or at a store. What type of information is included on the label?

8. List two prescription drugs that are exempt from child-resistant packaging.

9. Discuss the difference between prescription drug inserts for prescribers and for patients.

10. Using your favorite Internet search engine (Google, Yahoo, etc.), locate your State Board of Pharmacy web page and find your state pharmacy laws and regulations that govern pharmacy technicians, including permitted functions and the requirements for pharmacy technician registration or licensure. Does your state require certification, registration, or licensure for pharmacy technicians?

Alphabet Soup

There are many acronyms used in the medical profession. Fill in the full name of each acronym below.

a. HIPAA

b. DEA

c. FDA

d. NDA

e. ANDA

f. DAW

g. DNS

h. NABP

i. OTC

j. CMEA

k. CMI

l. PPI

m. PHI

n. NACDS

Word Search

```
B H M D A I O I T A C I L P P A G U R D W E N T D
A T L R B R I E T T I R W S A E S N E P S I D E P
W T S U B E T N O P S E D I D L D I I T I A T F N
N R I G R E I O E T I O E A S I A A D U E U A T I
E U R E E N S I A W M T F C E E N I C A T N E I D
D I T N V I I T I I D S F S N N A T D I H D L N O
I N C F I O O A I D R R T O T M I E T N B I N I C
T O A O A T I M C P B I U R T P A S C P C T S T T
A I C R T A T R O R R U N G R C B T V L L T N H
C T I C E M A O N O N G T G A U U E I A D T N U S
T A M E D R M F S T I O I E S P V T R I A F S I S
T M E M N O R N U E E T V T N A P N N I M I N A I
I R D E E F O I M C R O O E H E A L T A C E D M P
N O I N W N F E E T R N E C R O U W I E A T M I C
M F P T D I N N R E O I E N I T P T N C A T I T N
C N E A R H I I M D H M F T A I H U T O A O E E G
T I E D U L E C E H E O E E E M M E E T T T S D N
N H N M G A N I D E E K T M T O B E C E D U I R N
E T I I A E I D I A C N I E T E I U T O T O C O I
T L M N P H C E C L C S E T F T I P B I U O R A N
T A A I P D I M I T U H R N A I R H T I F N M N S
I E T S L E D R N H N E E A E G O B I N N O T B E
R H E T I T E E E I T E E I O T U E I C E R P N S
W D H R C C M M N N I U D I O S M T E A T C G P S
S E P A A E R U F F B H A U T O D C A C A M E F H
A T M T T T E S O O M R E O D T I C A P A N T R T
E C A I I O M N R R A I N V I C N A A E T E M E T
S E H O O R U O M M G O C V K D P O I E N R H I E
N T T N N P S C A A D O E P O U I R E I E A A I P
E O E K T O N I T T D O N O T S U B S T I T U T O
P R M B I T O U I R V N O S A M R C V N V D O T D
S P T I N E C T O V E R T H E C O U N T E R T K R
I D A P A T I E N T P A C K A G E I N S E R D O N
D I B N F O O D D R U G A D M I N I S T R A T I S
A E M F O O D D R U G A D M I N I S T R A T I O N
E I O T R E S N I E G A K C A P T N E I T A P O E
E N C N R W N E E R T T U A P I M I R A R I U R C
```

ABBREVIATEDNEWDRUGAPPLICATION
COMBATMETHAMPHETAMINEEPIDEMICACT
CONSUMERMEDICINEINFORMATION
DISPENSEASWRITTEN
DONOTSUBSTITUTE
DRUGENFORCEMENTADMINISTRATION

FOODDRUGADMINISTRATION
NEWDRUGAPPLICATION
OVERTHECOUNTER
PATIENTPACKAGEINSERT
PROTECTEDHEALTHINFORMATION

Chapter 3

Community and Ambulatory Care Pharmacy Practice

Learning Outcomes

This chapter reinforces the following learning outcomes discussed in Chapter 3/ Community and Ambulatory Care Pharmacy Practice of the *Manual for Pharmacy Technicians, 4th edition.*

- Describe the history of community and ambulatory care pharmacy practices.
- Describe the differences among the various types of practice sites in community and ambulatory care pharmacy practice.
- Describe the importance of the pharmacy technician's role in communicating with patients in the community and ambulatory care pharmacy settings.
- Explain the various steps and responsibilities involved in filling a prescription.
- Identify the trends in community and ambulatory care pharmacy practices.
- Describe the evolving role of the pharmacy technician in community and ambulatory care pharmacy practices.

Multiple Choice 14

Matching 14

True or False 15

Fill in the Blank 15

Short Answer 16

Alphabet Soup 16

Crossword Puzzle 17

Word Search 18

Multiple Choice

1. A bothersome or unwanted effect that results from the use of a drug, unrelated to the intended effect of the drug is a(an):

   a. Ill effect.
   b. Drug interaction.
   c. Adverse drug reaction.
   d. Toxic effect.

2. An ambulatory pharmacy is a pharmacy that:

   a. Only serves hospitalized patients.
   b. Travels to neighborhoods to provide services.
   c. Only serves patients who walk in or who have medications mailed to them.
   d. Only serves patients who need their medications compounded.

3. The portion of the cost of a prescription that the patient is responsible for paying, when a part of the cost is covered by a third-party payer, is a:

   a. Dispensing fee.
   b. Formulary charge.
   c. Ingredient cost.
   d. Copayment.

4. The term for the patient information approved by the FDA to help patients understand and use medication correctly is:

   a. Package insert.
   b. Prospective Drug Utilization Review pamphlet.
   c. Medication Guide.
   d. HIPAA Guide.

5. The legislation that precisely defined the guidelines for prescription drugs and established two categories of drugs is the:

   a. Durham-Humphrey Amendment.
   b. Food, Drug, and Cosmetic Act.
   c. Omnibus Budget Reconciliation Act.
   d. Health Insurance Portability and Accountability Act.

6. The legislation that most significantly changed the pharmacists' role in pharmacy practice is the:

   a. Durham-Humphrey Amendment.
   b. Food, Drug, and Cosmetic Act.
   c. Omnibus Budget Reconciliation Act.
   d. Health Insurance Portability and Accountability Act.

7. The legislation that most significantly changed the technicians' role in pharmacy practice is the:

   a. Durham-Humphrey Amendment.
   b. Food, Drug, and Cosmetic Act.
   c. Omnibus Budget Reconciliation Act.
   d. Health Insurance Portability and Accountability Act.

8. The legislation that protects individuals' private health information is the:

   a. Durham-Humphrey Amendment.
   b. Food, Drug, and Cosmetic Act.
   c. Omnibus Budget Reconciliation Act.
   d. Health Insurance Portability and Accountability Act.

9. When a patient is bringing a prescription to you for the first time, which of the following information is not necessary for the pharmacy to have?

   a. Correct spelling of name.
   b. Address and phone number(s).
   c. Marital status.
   d. Date of birth.

10. Examples of sources of third-party payers include:

    a. Government employers.
    b. Government programs such as Medicaid.
    c. Private insurance companies.
    d. All of the above.

Matching

Match the following medications with the appropriate REMS program. (Not all medication names will be used.)

A. alosetron (Lotronex)

B. clozapine (Clozaril, Fazaclo)

C. isotretinoin (Accutane, Amnesteem, Claravis, Sotret)

D. thalidomide (Thalomid)

E. dofetilide (Tikosyn)

_____ 1. iPledge Program

_____ 2. T.I.P.S. Program

_____ 3. PPL

_____ 4. S.T.E.P.S. Program

True or False

_____ 1. An adverse drug reaction is a bothersome or unwanted effect that results from the use of a drug, unrelated to the intended effect of the drug.

_____ 2. A generic drug is one that is covered by a patent and is, therefore, only available from a single manufacturer.

_____ 3. The Health Insurance Portability and Accountability Act (HIPAA) is legislation enacted by states to establish guidelines for the protection of patients' private health information.

_____ 4. A legend drug is one that, based on safety and potential for addiction, requires authorization from an authorized prescriber before a pharmacist can prepare and dispense the product.

_____ 5. The foundation of medication therapy management by pharmacists is the proper handling and preparation of the actual drug product by technicians.

_____ 6. Resolving third-party payer issues is a complicated task usually handled by pharmacists.

_____ 7. If an interaction with a patient seems to be escalating toward confrontation, it is best for the technician to involve another technician.

_____ 8. In order to maintain standard workflow, prescriptions should be processed in the order they are received.

_____ 9. The use of both isotretinoin and thalidomide is restricted because both medications can cause serious birth defects.

_____ 10. Counting devices use a scale to count units based on their weight or light beams to count units as they are poured through a machine.

_____ 11. The purpose of obtaining patients' signatures is to confirm that they have received the Medication Guides as required by the FDA.

_____ 12. A pharmacist generally completes special training to become certified to provide disease state management.

Fill in the Blank

1. The Durham-Humphrey Amendment to the Food, Drug and Cosmetic Act established two categories of drugs. These two categories are _____ drugs and _____ drugs.

2. Pharmaceutical care essentially encourages the establishment of the _____ as the manager of a patient's drug therapy.

3. _____ pharmacies are those where companies own a large number of pharmacies that all use the same name and logo and carry similarly branded OTC products.

4. _____ pharmacies are generally owned and staffed by one or two individuals.

5. The _____ regulates generic drugs so that they are equivalent in quality to corresponding brand-name drugs.

6. A _____ may require registration and other specific action by the physician, pharmacist, and patient before the medication can be dispensed.

7. The restricted-use drug used to treat patients with schizophrenia, _____, can cause a serious drop in white blood cells, so careful monitoring of these levels must be done regularly based on the patient's condition and medical history.

8. If the patient has prescription coverage by a third-party payer, the _____ is the amount of the cost of the prescription that the patient is responsible for paying.

9. A _____ is a list of drugs and their tiers that a specific third-party payer will cover.

10. Most third-party claims are now handled by _____, which are companies that contract with multiple third-party payers to process transactions and help establish and enforce their formularies.

11. The FDA requires some drugs to be dispensed with _____, which help patients avoid serious adverse events, inform them about known serious side effects, and provide directions for use to promote adherence to the treatment.

12. A product's _____ _____ can be used as a double check for technicians to make sure the correct drug product has been selected for filling.

Short Answer

1. Describe the differences among the various types of practice sites in community and ambulatory care pharmacy practice.

2. Explain the various steps and responsibilities involved in filling a prescription.

3. How has OBRA '90 affected pharmacy practice and, specifically, the practice of pharmacy technicians?

4. List five technician job responsibilities and discuss how one differentiates pharmacist duties from pharmacy technician duties.

5. When a patient is bringing a prescription to your pharmacy for the first time, what types of information are important to gather and why?

6. Discuss the five restricted-use medications that require Risk Evaluation and Mitigation Strategies (REMS). Include information about the purpose of the medications, the dangers to the patient, and the restrictions imposed.

7. Discuss the important aspects involved in point-of-sale (POS) transactions.

8. How could a pharmacy technician assist a pharmacist in accomplishing the three functions required of pharmacists by the Omnibus Budget Reconciliation Act (OBRA) filling a prescription for a Medicaid recipient?

9. List three newer practice trends pharmacies are using to serve their patients while also generating revenue. How would pharmacy technicians assist with these trends?

10. Discuss how pharmacists assist with disease state management.

Alphabet Soup

The following acronyms were used in Chapter 3. Fill in the full name of each acronym below.

a. DUR

b. OBRA

c. OTC

d. PBM

e. NDC

f. HMO

g. HIPAA

h. FDCA

i. REMS

j. IBS

k. NSAIDS

l. POS

m. DEA

Crossword Puzzle

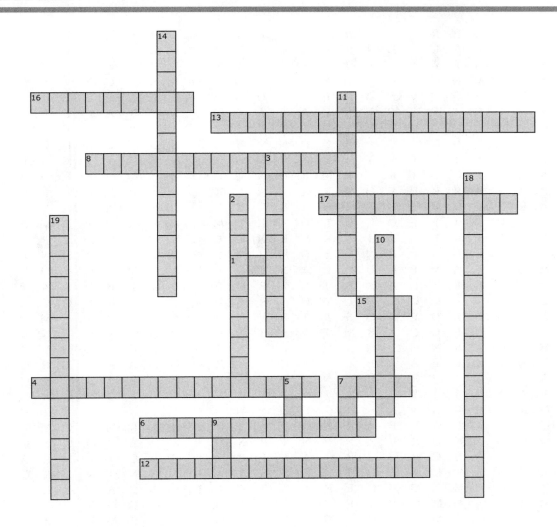

Across:

1. Companies that contract with third-party payers to process transactions
4. A unique number assigned to each drug, strength, and package size
6. A pharmacy that is part of corporately owned pharmacies
7. Lead to change in pharmacists' practice
8. A bothersome or unwanted drug effect
12. FDA-approved patient information for specific drugs
13. A pharmacy that provides medication services to walk-in patients
15. Managed care
16. A drug name that is covered by a patent
17. A drug name that is no longer covered by a patent

Down:

2. The preparation of a medication for a patient
3. The portion of the cost of a prescription that an insured patient pays
5. Pharmacist's screen of appropriateness of medication
7. Meds not requiring prescription
9. Identifier of medication
10. A list of drugs that a third-party payer will cover
11. The act of educating a patient about medication
14. Money collected from a third-party payer to cover cost of a prescription
18. Effects caused by the combined actions of two or more drugs
19. A pharmacy located in a medical center

Word Search

```
I  C  B  O  B  R  E  A  D  V  E  R  S  E  R  E  A  C  T  H  M  N  U  S  A
G  C  P  R  N  U  N  D  R  R  U  H  R  G  Y  R  V  U  D  E  O  O  P  S  C
N  G  S  A  E  A  N  A  E  I  A  R  M  P  T  R  R  D  I  H  S  O  B  N  N
N  C  T  M  N  E  D  O  N  E  S  B  U  A  C  C  O  B  R  A  C  T  Y  A  N
N  Y  I  I  E  U  M  N  B  A  E  N  N  D  D  E  A  L  E  C  C  C  E  A  H
I  C  T  D  A  E  H  P  E  N  C  A  E  A  S  M  E  R  M  Y  A  A  E  P  R
R  D  C  A  M  C  R  R  R  V  M  D  C  P  I  Y  I  S  A  R  D  E  E  I  N
A  G  A  B  N  O  I  H  P  A  S  D  N  M  S  O  F  S  N  E  F  R  D  H  S
E  D  E  M  T  N  E  M  Y  A  P  O  C  G  G  I  U  N  D  I  Y  E  M  B  P
S  A  R  E  D  O  T  R  T  P  M  R  U  N  A  E  D  O  N  M  U  S  R  G  A
R  A  E  A  R  R  H  E  O  H  R  R  I  A  L  R  L  A  A  B  N  R  E  L  U
A  D  S  E  M  P  S  G  S  C  D  L  S  O  I  E  O  C  R  U  A  O  A  Y  E
P  R  R  P  I  E  E  O  N  C  E  D  A  E  P  M  O  H  B  R  M  V  E  M  A
N  U  E  M  R  E  S  F  I  S  R  M  R  N  C  E  O  R  M  S  H  D  L  P  U
G  O  V  C  D  N  P  R  N  Y  L  U  M  R  O  F  F  Y  C  E  L  A  D  N  E
M  B  D  E  A  M  E  U  U  C  L  I  N  I  C  P  H  A  R  M  A  C  Y  O  B
D  R  A  E  P  N  O  A  S  B  I  L  E  B  G  E  C  E  I  E  B  D  S  A  Y
I  A  G  M  E  C  C  I  A  L  M  O  N  R  E  F  R  T  D  N  D  P  O  C  A
C  N  A  G  E  D  E  P  O  S  P  I  P  V  R  Y  U  P  O  T  M  Y  E  M  D
O  N  N  D  F  D  C  A  S  M  T  I  E  I  N  H  I  O  O  I  R  C  E  N  R
M  A  C  A  V  N  G  L  G  N  H  C  E  R  N  I  N  E  C  G  A  R  M  Y  S
Y  M  L  H  P  E  A  I  E  P  N  M  C  F  O  R  M  U  L  A  R  Y  T  H  C
A  E  R  E  A  P  R  M  E  T  N  E  M  E  S  R  U  B  M  E  I  R  O  T  G
P  A  A  N  I  I  Y  S  L  A  I  M  G  N  I  S  N  I  P  S  I  D  G  S  N
O  R  R  H  F  A  N  N  E  R  C  E  O  N  M  G  N  I  S  N  E  P  S  I  D
C  N  N  I  P  A  R  P  A  R  N  C  H  A  I  N  P  H  A  R  M  A  C  Y  U
O  U  M  A  N  U  R  E  A  N  E  N  T  R  S  M  P  B  H  A  B  P  C  N  O
P  E  C  G  B  C  R  M  C  R  C  A  N  E  C  M  A  G  P  C  I  A  N  R  A
A  C  D  S  R  C  A  A  O  I  M  S  C  S  Y  A  F  F  A  N  I  R  E  R  C
Y  S  R  H  H  E  M  M  C  L  N  A  A  T  U  A  F  S  A  C  A  M  I  C  R
M  S  O  N  O  M  C  N  I  E  U  I  C  R  I  H  A  N  C  O  G  T  O  T  C
E  Y  E  C  I  M  O  R  O  R  M  R  C  Y  O  O  R  V  S  R  M  E  P  I  P
C  N  D  N  E  N  M  O  L  U  N  M  Y  R  C  B  N  E  I  E  L  R  I  S  P
B  R  A  N  D  N  T  C  H  D  E  U  M  C  U  O  N  S  I  L  I  N  G  O  F
R  Y  O  C  A  A  M  R  A  H  P  N  I  A  H  C  M  I  A  A  O  D  U  U  R
T  E  C  R  R  I  M  N  R  O  P  P  I  H  A  M  A  S  R  C  A  D  R  L  C
```

ADVERSEREACTION

BRANDNAME

CHAINPHARMACY

CLINICPHARMACY

COPAYMENT

COUNSELING

DEA

DISPENSING

DUR

FDCA

FORMULARY

GENERICDRUG

HIPAA

HMO

NDC

OBRA

OTC

PBM

POS

REIMBURSEMENT

REMS

Chapter 4

Hospital Pharmacy Practice

Learning Outcomes

This chapter reinforces the following learning outcomes discussed in Chapter 4/ Hospital Pharmacy Practice of the *Manual for Pharmacy Technicians, 4th edition.*

- Describe the differences between centralized and decentralized pharmacies.
- List at least two types of services that are provided by hospital pharmacy departments.
- Explain how pharmacy policy and procedure manuals help technicians function efficiently with a large number of duties, responsibilities, and situations.
- List at least three different methods of drug distribution in which technicians play an active role.
- List the components of—and the role the technician has in—the medication management process.
- Describe the role accrediting and regulatory agencies play in a hospital pharmacy.
- List two types of technology that a pharmacy technician will work with in a hospital pharmacy.
- Describe quality control and quality improvement programs, including how they are used in hospital pharmacy practice.
- List at least three organizations that are involved with patient safety.
- Describe the financial impact that third-party payers have on hospitals.

Multiple Choice 20

Matching 20

True or False 21

Fill in the Blank 22

Short Answer 22

Alphabet Soup 22

Word Search 23

Multiple Choice

1. A system in which all medications are available for a prescriber to use on his or her patient is a(an):

    a. Closed formulary.
    b. Open formulary.
    c. Unit dose distribution system.
    d. Investigational drug program.

2. Historically, pharmacy services were:

    a. Primarily involved with drug distribution.
    b. Performed from a central pharmacy, usually in the basement.
    c. Provided medications in bulk containers to nursing units.
    d. All of the above.

3. Typically, in hospital organizations:

    a. The board of directors reports to the CEO.
    b. The CEO reports to the COO.
    c. The CFO reports to the board of directors.
    d. The COO reports to the CEO.

4. Technician responsibilities in a central pharmacy include all of the following *except*:

    a. Preparing IV antibiotics.
    b. Preparing IV chemotherapeutic agents.
    c. Performing functions related to quality control and quality improvement.
    d. Monitoring and evaluating patient response to medications.

5. The disadvantage of decentralized pharmacies is that:

    a. They require additional resources.
    b. They do not have as many filling stations as the central pharmacy.
    c. They are often located in the basement.
    d. The pharmacist has fewer opportunities to discuss the plan of care, answer drug information questions, and make appropriate drug therapy recommendations.

6. Pharmacy technicians are being used to help pharmacists in all of the following areas *except*:

    a. Collecting routine clinical data.
    b. Providing patient education.
    c. Tracking medication errors.
    d. Taking on management tasks.

7. For the manual process of filling medication carts or cassettes:

    a. Each medication is assigned to a drawer.
    b. Each patient is assigned to a drawer.
    c. Fill lists are generated to provide medications for 8 hours.
    d. Drawers contain drug information.

8. The pharmaceutical care model allows for new roles for the technician, which might include:

    a. Recording laboratory results in the pharmacist's patient database.
    b. Pharmacokinetic dosing.
    c. Infectious disease consultations.
    d. Drug information services.

Matching

Match the following terms with the appropriate descriptions.

A. Decentralized pharmacy services

B. Pharmacy satellites

C. Pharmacy and Therapeutics (P&T) Committee

D. Clinical pharmacy services

E. Investigational drug services

F. Drug distribution services

G. Medication management

H. Medication-use evaluation

I. Quality Improvement

J. Quality Control

_____ 1. Services provided by a pharmacist focused on patient care services to ensure that each medication is appropriate, safe, and cost effective (based on the diagnosis of the patient).

_____ 2. Pharmacy services that are provided on or near a patient care area, often supported by a central pharmacy.

_____ 3. A service that supports clinical trials involving medications where medications must be stored in a separate section of the pharmacy with limited access.

_____ 4. The system that begins when the medication is received by the pharmacy and ends when the medication is administered to the patient.

_____ 5. A physical space located in or near a patient care area that can provide a variety of distributive and clinical services.

_____ 6. A formal or systematic approach to analyzing the performance of a system or process.

_____ 7. A process of checks and balances (or procedures) that are followed during the provision of a service to ensure that the end services meet or exceed specified standards.

_____ 8. The group of processes that are included as Joint Commission standards and involve the entire medication use process, including selection, procurement of drugs, storage, prescribing, preparation and dispensing, administration, monitoring the effects of the medication, and evaluation of the effectiveness of the entire system.

_____ 9. A performance improvement method that evaluates how medications are being utilized to treat patients in the hospital, with the goal of improving medication use and optimizing patient therapy.

_____ 10. A group that meets on a routine basis to make decisions about the care of patients, with a focus on the safe and effective use of medications.

True or False

_____ 1. Pharmacy technicians may be assigned to management or lead responsibilities.

_____ 2. The advantage of centralized services is that a pharmacist also has more opportunities to discuss the plan of care, answer drug information questions, and make appropriate drug therapy recommendations with other health care providers.

_____ 3. The advantage of having technicians in decentralized pharmacies is that the technicians can respond quickly to any problems with medication storage cabinets.

_____ 4. Pharmacy technicians are not usually asked to participate on hospital committees because they do not perform tasks requiring clinical judgment.

_____ 5. An example of an ad hoc committee is the P&T Committee.

_____ 6. Pharmacists have the responsibility to operate and maintain automated drug distribution systems because pharmacists are licensed.

_____ 7. Every hospital pharmacy is required by The Joint Commission to maintain a policy and procedure manual.

_____ 8. Studies have shown that technicians are not as accurate at checking medication carts as pharmacists.

_____ 9. Technicians can screen medication orders for non-formulary status or identify if the medication is on the hospital's restricted list based on its high cost, high toxicity, or potential for over-prescribing.

_____ 10. Before a study is approved to be conducted in the hospital, a study protocol is developed, reviewed, and approved by the Joint Commission (TJC).

_____ 11. All medication storage areas in the hospital are assigned to be inspected at least monthly by pharmacy technicians.

_____ 12. When prescribers enter the order electronically, it is not necessary for a pharmacist to review the order for appropriateness.

Fill in the Blank

1. The _____ is an approved list of medications that are routinely stocked in the hospital pharmacy to treat the types of patients the hospital typically serves.

2. The_____ is at the top of the pharmacy department hierarchy in terms of management.

3. A pharmacy satellite is an example of a(an) _____ pharmacy service.

4. Every hospital pharmacy is required by The Joint Commission to maintain a _____ _____ _____ manual.

5. When a drug is administered to the patient, the dose is documented as given in the patient's _____ _____ _____.

6. The standing committee called the _____ _____ _____ _____ establishes a hospital formulary based on criteria such as indications for use, effectiveness, drug interactions, potential for errors and abuse, adverse effects, and cost.

7. Hospitals that typically only have a few drugs in a specific class of medications operate with a _____ formulary, which means that the list of available drugs is limited.

8. The hospital department that is responsible for the appropriate inspection of all medication storage areas to ensure that medications have not expired is the _____ department.

9. One of the most recognized accrediting agencies for hospitals is the _____ _____ _____.

10. Baxa Micromix® and Automix® machines are examples of _____ compounders.

11. Cardinal's Pyxis Medstation®, OmniCell's Single-Pointe™, and McKesson's ROBOTRx® are examples of _____ medication dispensing systems.

12. Quality improvement procedures can be prospective to identify system problems before they occur, such as a _____, or retrospective after a problem has occurred, such as _____. Both are systematic approaches with the goal of improving care to patients.

Short Answer

1. Describe the differences between centralized and decentralized pharmacies.

2. Explain the difference between a closed formulary and an open formulary.

3. What are the criteria used for the P&T Committee to make formulary decisions?

4. What is the procedure for receiving a verbal medication order?

5. Describe a procedure for prospective order review for hospitals where the pharmacy is not staffed 24 hours per day.

6. Describe the elements on a medication label intended for patient administration.

7. Explain the process of using bar codes for safe medication administration.

8. What is the purpose of MUEs?

9. What is the benefit of accreditation of hospitals?

10. What is the difference between Quality Improvement and Quality Control?

Alphabet Soup

The following acronyms were used in Chapter 4. Fill in the full name of each acronym below.

a. QC

b. QI

c. CQI

d. TQM

e. FMEA

f. RCA

g. ISMP

h. ASHP

i. IHI

j. TJC

k. IOM

l. AHRQ

m. CMS

n. NCQA

o. HMO

p. P&T Committee

q. MAR

r. MUE

s. IV

t. CEO

u. COO

v. CPOE

w. IRB

Word Search

```
A M E D I C A T I O N M A N A G E M E D Y M T I L
T N I L O R T N O C Y T I L A U Q L V R A N N T C
M R E Y R I R A I E I A C N M Q A N A I D O E L D
R A N L Z C E A S T U E I M I C Z L E E V I M O T
D H T O M E C O M N V O C M E E U O Z G O S E C D
L M L A I R D O S C I Z T N A M R I L I M S G O T
A L S P E T E E Q Y I G I R R D L T Z A A I A D O
N E R C I I T Y S L J L D O C A R L L N M M N S N
O E C N G A L M A A C L F M R N A N G T T M A A M
I L U T I E O R E A D D U T T I Y R F C M O M T M
T N E Y N I T I T I E T N T P R N C J R M C N E E
A N E U T N A A D S O E I T N T L I T C I T I L N
G N N T E E M I O C C L C N A U N M U G P N O L C
I L E C T C C L C E A L H E U L Y L A R A I T I P
T A I C A N C N D M T A Q N N I T T R O P O A T M
S L D O I T T O M D A N R R F T E A R O E J C I O
E E D D E N E C E H U L I Q I N R N E U T D I P O
V R E I N O I I T A T N N L P E T A N E A A D H O
N T L T T E R L M E M R L A N O N C L E V I E A M
I L E E M N I Q C O O G P L O N E L A I Q N M R L
N O N F O R M U L A R Y D R U G M N C V Z V T M Y
R T E M E N I L Y C A M R A H P E T I L L E T A S
E Q O A N Z L C L I N I C A L A G F M I E S D C L
I A N E M E V O R P M I Y T I L A U Q D A T T Y O
R A A T E E I L A R T N E C E D N L T U E I I M E
N I R Z T I A E O L I L R A D T A E O A R G S I S
T C L O S I D F O R M U L A R Y M M E O I A S I A
Q U A L I T Y I M P R O V E M E N T I S O T I R T
D T R T N O C Y T I L A U Q M N O I A E U I M O Z
U N I T D O S U U E D D I A Q M I E O I I O M R T
C N N O I S S I M M O T N I O J T O Y E T N O Y U
N O N F O R M U L A R Y D R U M A Z Z I O A C A D
T Z D L E O F H R O L I C C Q R C T I Y M L T T G
S A T E L L I T E P H A R M A A I Y L D S D N M I
C Y A M S E I E A Y I I N L Y C D C M E I R I C R
C L D E C E N T A L I Z E D T M E N R A E U O D R
N A S D I A C S C E N E T R T D M P I O P G J T I
```

CENTRALIZED
CLINICAL
CLOSEDFORMULARY
DECENTRALIZED
INVESTIGATIONALDRUG
JOINTCOMMISSION

MEDICATIONMANAGEMENT
NONFORMULARYDRUG
QUALITYCONTROL
QUALITYIMPROVEMENT
SATELLITEPHARMACY
UNITDOSE

Chapter 5

Home Care Pharmacy Practice

Learning Outcomes

This chapter reinforces the following learning outcomes discussed in Chapter 5/ Home Care Pharmacy Practice of the *Manual for Pharmacy Technicians, 4th edition*.

- Identify the historical reasons for establishing home care services and the growth of the home care industry.
- Cite the seven goals of home care therapy.
- Identify the members of the home care team and describe their primary roles in the home care process.
- Identify the most common diseases or conditions treated with home care services.
- Identify the top drug classes used in home infusion therapy. List one or two parameters for these drugs that affect how they are used in the home environment.
- Compare the advantages and disadvantages of the types of infusion systems available for use in a patient's home.
- List the labeling requirements for sterile products that are to be used in a patient's home.
- Outline the factors that are important to consider when determining expiration dates for sterile products used in the home care setting.

Multiple Choice 26

Matching 27

True or False 27

Fill in the Blank 28

Short Answer 28

Crossword Puzzle 29

Word Search 30

Multiple Choice

1. Home infusion has become popular because:

   a. It is cost-effective.
   b. Patients may avoid infections originating from hospital stays.
   c. Patients can continue with fairly normal lives.
   d. All of the above.

2. The decision to accept or refuse the referral for home care therapy is based upon:

   a. The ability and willingness of the patient or the caregivers to perform the tasks required to administer therapy at home.
   b. The appropriateness and feasibility of the therapeutic plan.
   c. The assurance that home care therapy will not place too much of a financial burden on the patient or the home infusion company.
   d. All of the above.

3. In the home care environment, maintenance of intravenous catheters is the sole responsibility of the:

   a. Physician.
   b. Pharmacist.
   c. Patient or caregiver.
   d. Nurse.

4. Pharmacy technicians are responsible for:

   a. Compounding, preparing, and labeling medications.
   b. Maintaining the compounding room and drug storage areas.
   c. Coordinating of the IV room.
   d. All of the above.

5. In general, antibiotics are chosen based on:

   a. The stability of the antibiotic.
   b. The organism(s) identified in the cultures.
   c. The route of administration.
   d. The cost.

6. Cephalosporins are very easy to use in home care because:

   a. They have a low incidence of adverse reactions and require minimal monitoring.
   b. They are stable for 10 days after admixture.
   c. Most can be administered as IV push.
   d. All of the above.
   e. None of the above.

7. Penicillins are a common IV antibiotic used in the home because:

   a. They have a low incidence of adverse reactions and require minimal monitoring.
   b. They are stable for 10 days after admixture.
   c. They can be given once a day.
   d. All of the above.
   e. None of the above.

8. Due to reactions to amphotericin infusions, patients may be premedicated with:

   a. Oral acetaminophen and diphenhydramine.
   b. Normal saline.
   c. Dextrose 5% syringes.
   d. Heparin.

9. A therapy often added to offset bone marrow toxicity is:

   a. Foscarnet.
   b. Filgrastim.
   c. Ganciclovir.
   d. None of the above.

10. Patients receiving parenteral nutrition require intensive monitoring, which usually includes weekly:

   a. Laboratory tests.
   b. Fluid status.
   c. Weights.
   d. All of the above.

Matching

Matching I

Match the following terms with the appropriate descriptions.

A. AIDS-related infections

B. Osteomyelitis

C. Septic arthritis

D. Cellulitis

E. Endocarditis

_____ 1. Infection of the tissue that lines the joints (synovium).

_____ 2. Acute inflammatory infection of the skin that often extends deep into the subcutaneous tissue (tissue under the skin).

_____ 3. Infection that occurs when bacteria (e.g., staphylococcus aureus) invades bone.

_____ 4. Infection of the heart valves or heart tissue.

_____ 5. Fungal Infections, Viral Infections, Cytomegalovirus (CMV).

Matching II

Match the following medications with the correct drug class.

A. Cipro

B. Vancomycin

C. Primaxin

D. Ancef

E. Amphotericin B

F. Foscarnet

G. Unasyn

_____ 1. Cephalosporins

_____ 2. Penicillins

_____ 3. Fluoroquinolones

_____ 4. Carbapenems

_____ 5. Antifungals

_____ 6. Antivirals

_____ 7. Other

True or False

_____ 1. Patients first began receiving infusion therapy in the home, rather than in an institutional setting, in the late 1950s.

_____ 2. The major goal of home care pharmacy practice is to provide safe and effective infusion therapy in the home even if it costs much more than infusions given in the hospital.

_____ 3. An intake coordinator for home health care is usually a pharmacy technician.

_____ 4. It should only take a quick visit for the nurse to train the patient or caregiver about how to administer medications.

_____ 5. Anti-infectives account for the majority of pharmaceuticals used in home infusion therapy.

_____ 6. Red Man Syndrome is a reaction from rapid infusion of penicillin that causes a redness or flushing of the head and torso.

_____ 7. Normal saline, commonly used to flush the catheter before and after the infusion of medication, is incompatible with amphotericin B.

_____ 8. To avoid making parenteral nutrition bags that cannot be used, the technician should coordinate mixing of a patient's parenteral nutrition to follow scheduled laboratory blood draws and pharmacist and nursing assessments and visits.

_____ 9. Enteral nutrition is the intravenous administration of specialized formulas that are high in required nutrients.

_____ 10. Ninety percent of home care narcotic orders are for meperidine.

_____ 11. Most products prepared for use by home care patients fall into risk level 2 (medium risk) because they are stored for more than 7 days.

_____ 12. For drugs to be given via an ambulatory infusion device, at least 10-hour stability at room temperature or warmer is required.

Fill in the Blank

1. The leaking of intravenous solutions into areas outside of the vein, resulting in potentially severe tissue damage, is called _____.

2. When a caregiver treats all patients as if they were potentially infectious, he or she is taking _____ _____ to prevent exposure to human blood or other potentially infectious material.

3. An infusion pump equipped with IV medication error prevention software is called a _____ pump.

4. An intravenous administration system containing reservoirs that consist of multiple layers of stretchy, elastic-like membranes within a hard or soft shell is called a(n) _____ _____ _____.

5. A type of pain management in which the patient receives parenteral narcotics with a basal/continuous rate and/or has the capabilities to self-administer fixed bolus doses using an electronic ambulatory infusion pump is called _____ _____ _____.

6. Rocephin is a member of the _____ drug class of antibiotics.

7. The syndrome caused by infusing vancomycin too quickly is called _____ _____ _____.

8. Normal saline is incompatible with amphotericin B—mixing the two results in _____.

9. _____ _____ _____ is intravenous nutrition that provides a patient with all of the fluid and essential nutrients he or she needs when oral hydration is difficult or impossible.

10. USP chapter _____ is part of an educational/advisory section of the USP standards for aseptic compounding (sterile compounding).

11. Most products prepared for use by home care patients fall into risk level _____ because they are stored for more than 7 days.

12. A(n) _____ _____ _____ is a vertical flow hood specially designed for the safe preparation of cytotoxic and other hazardous drugs.

Short Answer

1. Discuss the reasons home infusion therapy has become popular.

2. Discuss the types of information that might be included in a care plan.

3. Identify the members of the home care team and describe their primary roles in the home care process.

4. Explain the difference between enteral feeding and parenteral nutrition therapy.

5. Discuss the various types of home infusion systems.

Crossword Puzzle

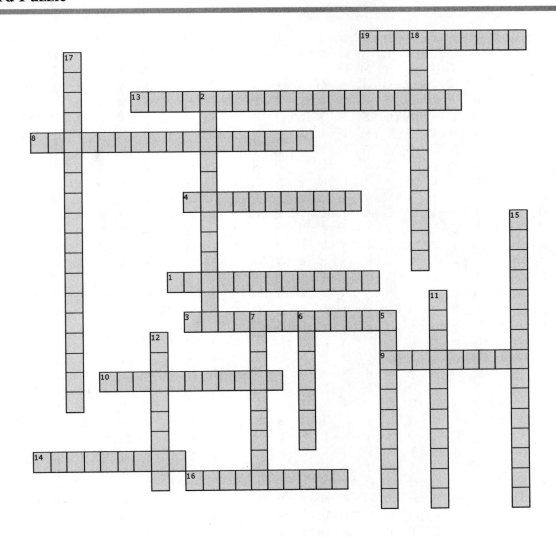

Across:

1. Leaking of intravenous solutions into areas outside of the vein
3. Infection of the bone
4. Mediator in home care process
8. Home care person who helps to set up the patient referral
9. An antiviral
10. Anti-infectives
13. Wearing personal protective equipment, hand washing
14. A cephalosporin
16. Administered by some means other than oral intake
19. Infection of the skin

Down:

2. Infection of the heart valves or heart tissue
5. Infusion pumps equipped with IV medication error prevention software
6. Nutrient delivery where fluid is given directly into the gastrointestinal tract
7. A penicillin
11. An antifungal
12. A carbapenem
15. Infection of the synovial tissue
17. Intravenous system for home infusions
18. A fluoroquinolone

Word Search

```
T A T S E R I A I N T A K E C O O R D I N A T O R
N E C I F M F L U O R O Q I U N O L A N E S I M I R I
E S E T I L E Y M O E T S O R E G A N A M E S A C
I U N I N A T O I A O I E X T A V A S A T I O N A L
B N I R O S L I C C N C E P A R E N T E R E L R L
S I C H E C A G S E S S T N A L U L U N F S O O T
A V S T O E G G M L L R N X D S O C I T N T H A U
E E I R S I N A A L E L E I R O P S O L A H P E C
T R S A P S U N R U L T U X R S C S C N T E T L S O
A S E C E C F A T L H P M L L O N A I T O S L S O
R A L I N E I M P I A A A A I I P D R S A A S E T
O L S T I P T E U T C U R L L T R S E D R I E L N
G P N P C H N S M I L I A L A O E N A E I C R A M
A R S E I A A A P I V R I N E E O S T L D T T E A
N E I S L L E C R I R C T C I L M N Y A A S I A L
A C T A L O R A T E I S O T O T E N I T S H N S P
M A I A E S C N T N A K I N E N T E R A L L P I S
E U L L N P A N E Q O D I D S P I T D A A P T E I
S T E O S O E P R T R U S A E I L L I C I N E P C
A I Y A E R L E N A Q S M A R T P U M P S R T A S
C O M L O I S O C O E N O I T A S A V A R T X E N
A N O C O N B O R N A C P A R E N T E R A L U S L
O S E A R S D O L O N I U Q O R O U L F L T M S A L
O I T L A N U N M S S E I S T I K P C I A E A R L
I T S S E L O A E U I I S S M C T A T N N C S P M
T I O I F T O R I L E N L N L E M M R E B T S F O L
A D I T A N T I F U N G A L I A N N P O O I E S L
S R C I O I A N T I V I R A L U R E E A N I E I O
A A E L A E N D O C A R D I T D B E P A C E N O X
V C T U A A L A M E N E P A B R A C V A X T D T I
A A O L A R O T F I E I S A A A A N T I B I O T T
R D S L A N T I B I O T I C S H U A A T T R A E U
T N N E S C E T O I B I T N A V X L I O I N A C A U
X E I C R N I L R T A M S L A G N U F I T N A C U
E P I T I D S O A I E A M A N I L C L N K T C D S
```

ANTIBIOTICS
ANTIFUNGALS
ANTIVIRALS
CARBAPENEMS
CASEMANAGER
CELLULITIS
CEPHALOSPORINS
ENDOCARDITIS
ENTERAL

EXTRAVASATION
FLUOROQUINOLONES
INTAKECOORDINATOR
OSTEOMYELITIS
PARENTERAL
PENICILLINS
SEPTICARTHRITIS
SMARTPUMPS
UNIVERSALPRECAUTIONS

Chapter 6

Specialty Pharmacy Practice

Learning Outcomes

This chapter reinforces the following learning outcomes discussed in Chapter 6/Specialty Pharmacy Practice of the *Manual for Pharmacy Technicians, 4th edition*.

- Describe the historic development of nuclear pharmacy practice.
- Explain the basic concepts of radioactivity and nuclear medicine as they relate to nuclear pharmacy practice.
- Explain the role of nuclear medicine and nuclear pharmacy in patient diagnosis and treatment.
- Describe the various aspects of nuclear pharmacy practice.
- Identify the common areas for technician involvement in the practice of nuclear pharmacy.
- Explain the role of pharmacy technicians in compounding specialties such as veterinary pharmacy practice.

Multiple Choice 32

Matching 33

True or False 33

Fill in the Blank 34

Short Answer 34

Internet Research 34

Multiple Choice

1. The function of nuclear medicine studies is used:

   a. To augment the anatomic information that is obtained by traditional imaging modalities.
   b. To treat certain diseases by destructive effects of certain types of radioactive emissions.
   c. Both a and b.
   d. None of the above.

2. The emission of radiation that is released from an unstable nucleus is called:

   a. Radioactive decay.
   b. Nuclear pharmacy.
   c. Radioactivity.
   d. Positron emission tomography.

3. Unique aspects of nuclear pharmacy operations include:

   a. Location of nuclear pharmacies.
   b. Workflow and staffing.
   c. Restricted and nonrestricted areas.
   d. Preparation and dispensing.
   e. All of the above.

4. Generally, because of the challenge of working with radioactivity, most pharmacies can only deliver final materials to hospitals within:

   a. A 2- or 3-hour travel distance from the pharmacy.
   b. The same city.
   c. A 30-minute travel distance from the pharmacy.
   d. An approved transportation company's routes instate.

5. Which of the following statements are true?

   a. Pets may take some types of human medications.
   b. Humans may take some types of veterinarian medications.
   c. A large-sized animal may require a smaller dose than a traditional house pet.
   d. The Society of Veterinary Hospital Pharmacists is an organization consisting of pharmacists who work exclusively at hospitals dedicated to the care of animals.

6. Radiopharmaceuticals are dispensed upon:

   a. The milligram (mg) amount of the product.
   b. The amount of radioactivity that will be administered to the patient.

7. Preparing radioactive pharmaceuticals by attaching radioactivity to a ligand is the job of a:

   a. Pharmacy technician.
   b. Radiologic technician.
   c. Radiologist.
   d. Pharmacist.

8. The area where white blood cells are isolated and radio-labeled must be:

   a. The biohazard risk of handling blood products.
   b. The restricted area due to the use of radioactive materials.
   c. A segregated area away from traffic to comply with sterile product compounding guidelines.
   d. All of the above.
   e. None of the above.

9. To prepare a radiopharmaceutical, a specified amount of the Tc-99m radioactive material is added to a(n):

   a. Gamma photon.
   b. Radiopharmaceutical kit.
   c. Positron emission tomography.
   d. IV injection.

10. Pharmacists who specialize in nuclear pharmacy are certified by the:

   a. BPS.
   b. NIH.
   c. USP.
   d. NRC.

Matching

Match the following terms with the appropriate descriptions.

A. restricted areas

B. half-life

C. hazardous material

D. positron emission tomography

E. ligand

F. nonrestricted areas

G. radioactive decay

H. NORM

_____ 1. Radioactivity that is present naturally in the environment.

_____ 2. The process of providing stability to an unstable nucleus by removing excess energy.

_____ 3. An advanced nuclear imaging technique that involves the use of short-lived radioactive materials to produce three-dimensional, colored images of those materials functioning in the body.

_____ 4. Areas of a nuclear pharmacy where radioactive materials are prohibited.

_____ 5. Chemical substance that will behave in a certain way when injected into the body.

_____ 6. Any material that poses a risk to people, animals, property, or the environment.

_____ 7. Areas of a nuclear pharmacy where radioactive materials are used and stored.

_____ 8. The amount of time required for one-half of the amount of radioactivity to decay.

True or False

_____ 1. The human body contains small amounts of radioactive carbon and potassium.

_____ 2. The functional information provided by nuclear medicine studies is used to augment the anatomic information that is obtained by traditional imaging modalities such as x-ray, computed tomography (CT), or magnetic resonance imaging (MRI).

_____ 3. Radiopharmaceuticals must be compounded on a weekly basis due to the radioactive component of the products.

_____ 4. The restricted areas are the general areas of the pharmacy where the staff and visitors can be assured of having limited to no contact with radioactive materials.

_____ 5. Very often, pharmacy technicians are responsible for maintaining appropriate recordkeeping and radioactive waste disposal.

_____ 6. When dispensing radiopharmaceuticals, the activity for the dose must be accurate at the time the material is dispensed.

_____ 7. After every product prepared is compounded, it undergoes quality control testing before any patient dose is released from the pharmacy.

_____ 8. Common quality control tests performed in a nuclear pharmacy require oversight of a nuclear medicine physician.

_____ 9. The sources of regulatory compliance involve the Nuclear Regulatory Commission (NRC) and the Department of Transportation (DOT).

_____ 10. Currently, pharmacist technicians are responsible for all aspects of the preparation and dispensing of radiopharmaceuticals used for therapeutic purposes.

_____ 11. The FDA "Orange Book" is a listing of all animal drug products that have been approved for safety and effectiveness.

_____ 12. A fairly innocuous drug used in the canine population (aspirin, for example) can be lethal to cats because they have a deficiency in the normal metabolic pathway for this drug.

Fill in the Blank

1. _____ _____ is an area of pharmacy practice that involves the preparation and dispensing of radioactive pharmaceutical products.

2. Another term for radioactive pharmaceutical products is _____.

3. A radioactive emission that occurs due to the elemental composition of the earth is called _____ gas, and it is a concern to many homeowners.

4. Radiopharmaceuticals are dispensed based on the amount of radioactivity that will be administered to the patient. An assay in nuclear pharmacy describes the number of _____ _____ per mL and is expressed as mCi/mL

5. A _____ _____ survey meter is a portable radiation detector that can be used to identify the presence of radioactive material and quantify the amount present at a particular location.

6. The _____ _____ is the most widely used piece of equipment and the most essential for the preparation and dispensing of radiopharmaceutical doses that will be administered to patients undergoing nuclear medicine studies.

7. The _____ _____ is used to quantify small amounts of radioactivity, to count samples and quantify the amount of radioactivity present at given locations in the pharmacy, and to identify what type of radioactive material is present in the sample.

8. The job of a radiopharmacist when preparing radioactive pharmaceuticals is to attach radioactivity to a _____.

9. The radionuclide generator system is designed to allow continual production of the radioisotope _____, which is used in most of the radiopharmaceutical products administered today.

10. Radiopharmaceuticals are most often dispensed as a(n)_____ _____, meaning one dose for one patient in one administration vessel.

11. The most substantial factor used to decrease radiation exposure to the radiation worker is _____.

12. The FDA _____ _____ is a listing of all animal drug products that have been approved for safety and effectiveness.

Short Answer

1. Describe the historic development of nuclear pharmacy practice.

2. Explain the basic concepts of radioactivity and nuclear medicine as they relate to nuclear pharmacy practice.

3. Explain the role of nuclear medicine and nuclear pharmacy in patient diagnosis and treatment.

4. Identify the common areas for technician involvement in the practice of nuclear pharmacy.

5. Explain the role of pharmacy technicians in compounding specialties such as veterinary pharmacy practice.

Internet Research

1. Perform an Internet search using "FDA" and "veterinary" or go to http://www.fda.gov/AnimalVeterinary/default.htm. When was this web page last updated?

2. What types of information are available? What types of information found here would be helpful in a pharmacy that compounds veterinary medication?

3. Perform an Internet search to locate nuclear pharmacy technician training programs. Choose a program and find out:

    a. Where it is located.
    b. Length of study.
    c. Approximate cost.
    d. Certificate offered?

Chapter 7

Drug Information Resources

Learning Outcomes

This chapter reinforces the following learning outcomes discussed in Chapter 7/ Drug Information Resources of the *Manual for Pharmacy Technicians, 4th edition*.

- Classify a drug information request.
- Explain how to obtain appropriate background information for a drug request.
- Distinguish between questions that may be answered by a technician and those that should be answered only by a pharmacist.
- Given a specific pharmacy-related question, identify the best resource to use to find the answer.
- Describe how to find answers to drug information questions at the workplace.

Multiple Choice 36

Matching 37

True or False 38

Fill in the Blank 38

Short Answer 39

Alphabet Soup 39

Internet Research 39

Multiple Choice

1. Indexing systems such as Medline, which provide a list of journal articles on the topic that is being searched, are referred to as:

   a. Primary references.
   b. Secondary references.
   c. Tertiary references.
   d. Dewey decimal systems.

2. You are asked how much a prescription will cost a patient. What are the considerations in answering this question?

   a. What is the cost of the medication?
   b. What is the mark-up or profit the pharmacy needs to make on the product?
   c. What type of insurance does the patient have and will it pay for all or a part of the prescription?
   d. All of the above.

3. If you notice a potentially dangerous situation such as a patient purchasing drugs with known serious interactions, you should:

   a. Not say anything because it is not in your scope of practice.
   b. Ask the pharmacist about the situation after the patient leaves the pharmacy to protect the patient's privacy.
   c. Make a note of the problem and turn it in to the pharmacist's supervisor.
   d. Ask the patient to wait a moment while you check on something, and then quietly check with the pharmacist before the patient makes the purchase and leaves the pharmacy.

4. As part of a systematic search strategy, a pharmacist is taught to:

   a. First consult primary references, then secondary references, and finally tertiary references.
   b. First consult tertiary references, then secondary references, and finally primary references.
   c. First consult tertiary references, then primary references, and finally secondary references.
   d. None of the above.

5. Which of the following are the most common references used because they are easy to use, convenient, readily accessible, concise, and compact?

   a. Primary references.
   b. Secondary references.
   c. Tertiary references.
   d. None of the above.

6. United States Pharmacopeia Drug Information (USPDI) (published by Thomson, Micromedex) is:

   a. A comprehensive reference system that is accessed electronically via Internet, CD-ROM, and PDA, and contains comprehensive drug information, Material Safety Data Sheets, patient information, and more.
   b. A detailed, comprehensive, general drug information reference, with complete drug monographs organized by therapeutic class, FDA- and nonFDA-approved uses of medications, and preparation and administration instructions for injectable products.
   c. An electronic drug information database that is widely used in retail chain pharmacies as well as pharmacy schools and hospitals and contains complete monographs for prescription and OTC drugs, dietary supplements and investigational drugs with indications (FDA-approved and off-label uses), pharmacology, pharmacokinetics, dosing and administration, drug interactions, warnings and precautions, pregnancy and lactation information, adverse effects, and available strengths with photos.
   d. A three-volume set that provides medication information for health care professionals and patients.

7. Questions regarding injectable drugs may concern:

   a. Concentrations.
   b. Admixture solutions.
   c. Infusion rates.
   d. All of the above.
   e. None of the above.

8. It may be assumed that medications listed as compatible under specific conditions:

   a. Will be compatible at higher concentration.
   b. Will be compatible in different solutions.
   c. Will be compatible for 24 hours.
   d. All of the above.
   e. None of the above.

9. A good reference for information on veterinary compounding and food ingredients, colorings, preservatives, and flavorings is:

   a. Trissel's Handbook on Injectable Drugs.
   b. King Guide to Parenteral Admixture.
   c. Extended Stability for Parenteral Drugs.
   d. USP Pharmacist's Pharmacopeia.

10. The most reliable reference for interactions between prescription medications and herbal remedies is:

    a. Facts and Comparisons.
    b. The Red Book.
    c. The Natural Medicines Comprehensive Database.
    d. USP Pharmacist's Pharmacopeia.

Matching

A. Pharmacist

B. Knowledgeable Pharmacy Technician

C. Debatable—give reasons

Indicate which of the pharmacy staff should answer the following questions, keeping in mind best utilization of resources:

_____ 1. What is the brand name of warfarin?

_____ 2. Do Naprosyn and Aleve contain the same active ingredient?

_____ 3. Who manufactures Enbrel?

_____ 4. Is Prilosec available as a generic? Is it a prescription or over-the-counter (OTC) product?

_____ 5. What dosage forms of Imitrex are available in your pharmacy?

_____ 6. Is Zoloft available as a liquid? If so, what size and concentration are available?

_____ 7. What are the prices of Adalat CC and Procardia XL?

_____ 8. How long is the shortage of albumin expected to last?

_____ 9. Should Lovenox be stored in the refrigerator?

_____ 10. How long is a flu shot stable after it is drawn up in a syringe?

_____ 11. How many milliliters are in an ounce?

_____ 12. How should ampicillin be reconstituted?

_____ 13. In what controlled substance schedule is zolpidem (Ambien)?

_____ 14. Can Tiazac be substituted for Cardizem CD (is it AB rated)?

_____ 15. How many times can a prescription be transferred from one store to another?

_____ 16. Where can I find the phone number for Sanofi Aventis?

_____ 17. When will the patent for Lipitor expire?

_____ 18. Where can I get more Lovenox teaching kits?

_____ 19. Where can I find the Vaccine Information Sheet for the influenza vaccine?

True or False

_____ 1. When you are asked a question about the usual dose of a medication, you may answer the question if you know the answer.

_____ 2. Consumers may not understand which questions a pharmacy technician can answer and which questions should be referred to the pharmacist.

_____ 3. The term "scope of practice" means any work you have been allowed to do in your work environment.

_____ 4. All drug information requests should be answered in written and referenced format.

_____ 5. When answering questions from patients, you will be more respected as an expert if you use medical terminology as much as possible.

_____ 6. If you have heard a pharmacist answer a clinical question many times, it is okay for you to give the answer you know that the pharmacist would have given?

_____ 7. Answers to many questions may be found in a multitude of references.

_____ 8. Many references are available in several formats such as "hard copy," online, or downloaded to computers or hand held devices.

_____ 9. If a physician's name is associated with Internet information, it is probably a reliable Internet site.

_____ 10. One of the most important steps in answering a drug information question is follow-up such as inquiries to the requestor about whether the information was useful and/or if it was answered. This will ensure that the response was complete.

_____ 11. The Red Book is a good source for lists of sugar, lactose, galactose, alcohol-free products, sulfite-containing products, and medications that shouldn't be crushed.

Fill in the Blank

1. A web-based searching system sponsored by the National Library of Medicine, which can be used to access Medline journal citations, is called _____.

2. An online database sponsored by the government, which contains health information for the public on over 500 health conditions, is called _____.

3. If a person wanted to compare the major side effects of all of the anti-psychotic medications, the best type of reference for finding this information would be a _____ reference.

4. All prescription medications provide an information sheet that contains general drug information, including indications, adverse effects, drug interactions, dosage forms, stability, and dosing information. This informational sheet is called a _____ _____.

5. The Drug Information Handbook, the Pediatric Dosage Handbook, the Drug Information Handbook for Oncology, the Geriatric Dosage Handbook, and the Drug Information Handbook for Psychiatry are all published by _____.

6. A reference called the _____ _____ contains product information and prices for prescription drugs, over-the-counter products, and medical supplies; NDC numbers for all products, available packaging, and therapeutic equivalence ratings; and a comprehensive listing of manufacturers, wholesalers, and third-party administrator directories.

7. A reference called the _____ _____ is used to determine if drugs are bioequivalent.

8. Vaccine Information Statements that explain the benefits and risks of vaccines can be found online at the _____ web site.

9. In case of poisoning or if over-exposure occurs, the _____ _____ _____ should be called at 1-800-222-1222.

10. The ___'s web site contains links for consumers and health care professionals regarding drug information such as new drug approvals, drug shortages, safety information, and generic drug bioequivalence (Orange Book).

Short Answer

1. When a request for drug information is made, what information should you gather from the requestor?

2. What are the classifications of drug information questions and why is it important to classify drug information questions?

3. Explain the terms "primary," "secondary," and "tertiary" references. Discuss the advantages and disadvantages of using primary, secondary, and tertiary references.

4. What does MSDS refer to and what is its purpose?

5. Information found on the Internet should always be evaluated for believability, the validity of the source, accuracy, supporting evidence, and timeliness. Describe how you would evaluate an Internet resource to ensure that it is a reliable source of information.

6. A customer comes into your pharmacy and has questions regarding side effects from the medication she purchased yesterday. The pharmacist is extremely busy and there is a line of patients waiting to speak to the pharmacist. You have a line of patients waiting to be checked out at the cash register. What should you do?

7. Explain why the PDR may not be as useful as other resources in comparing products.

Alphabet Soup

The following acronyms were used in Chapter 7. Fill in the full name of each acronym below.

a. CDC

b. NIH

c. CDER

d. FDA

e. AHFS DI

f. AJHP

g. JAPhA

h. ASHP

i. OTC

j. PDR

k. APhA

l. MSDS

m. AAPCC

n. NLM

o. ISMP

Internet Research

1. Conduct an Internet search to find out what vaccines are necessary for travel to Peru. What vaccines are needed?

2. Go to www.ashp.org and find out how a technician training program becomes accredited. What are the steps?

3. Go to www.ashp.org/shortage and list five shortages and when they might return to the market.

4. Go to www.ismp.org and list three strategies for error prevention highlighted on this site.

Chapter 8

Communication and Teamwork

Learning Outcomes

This chapter reinforces the following learning outcomes discussed in Chapter 8/ Communication and Teamwork of the *Manual for Pharmacy Technicians, 4th edition.*

- Describe the purpose of various types of communications that occur within pharmacy practice settings, including the role of the pharmacy technician.
- List the basic elements of verbal and nonverbal communications.
- Given a specific patient encounter scenario, compare and contrast effective and ineffective communication skills.
- Describe how to vary communication techniques to improve success when working with special patient populations.
- Identify the types of health care professionals with whom a pharmacy technician may communicate as well as effective strategies for those communications.
- Describe the types of behaviors that should be demonstrated by pharmacy technicians to promote effective working relationships with other health care team members.

Multiple Choice 42

Matching 43

True or False 43

Fill in the Blank 44

Short Answer 44

Word Search 45

Multiple Choice

1. A pharmacy technician is defined as:

   a. "An individual working in a pharmacy who can assist the pharmacist with all tasks."
   b. "An individual working in a pharmacy who, under the supervision of a licensed pharmacist, assists in pharmacy activities that do not require the professional judgment of a pharmacist."
   c. "An individual working in a pharmacy who, under the supervision of a licensed pharmacist, meets with patients and answers questions about medications."
   d. "An individual working in a pharmacy who operates the cash register and answers the phone."

2. Strong communication skills help to:

   a. Avoid misunderstandings.
   b. Avoid interpersonal conflicts.
   c. Ensure patient safety.
   d. All of the above.

3. Miscommunications in pharmacies could result in problems with:

   a. Inventory control.
   b. Licensure maintenance.
   c. Employment.
   d. All of the above.
   e. None of the above.

4. The goal of effective communication is to:

   a. Ensure that the recipient party hears the same message, both in content and intent, as the deliverer and that the intended result of that message is achieved.
   b. Ensure that the deliverer conveys to the recipient the required HIPAA information.
   c. Ensure that the recipient party understands the medication informational sheets.
   d. Ensure that the deliverer speaks the same language as the recipient.

5. Patients may display confrontational behavior due to:

   a. Acute illness.
   b. Uncontrolled pain.
   c. Terminal illness.
   d. All of the above.
   e. None of the above.

6. Since pharmacists are human beings just as patients are, pharmacists:

   a. May become angry with patients due to stressful work.
   b. May expect to be viewed as objects just as patients are.
   c. Can struggle with their personal lives and may share this with patients.
   d. Must manage personal feelings while recognizing and considering the feelings of their patients.

7. Interpersonal communication involves a complex array of processes focused on:

   a. Transmitting, receiving, and processing information.
   b. Talking, listening, and writing with others.
   c. E-mailing, twittering, and blogging.
   d. Listening, hearing, and analyzing information.

8. Professional behavior may include:

   a. Jokes.
   b. Political comments.
   c. Religious comments.
   d. All of the above.
   e. None of the above.

9. In a busy pharmacy, it is acceptable to:

   a. Take personal mobile phone calls.
   b. Text.
   c. Use Facebook.
   d. All of the above.
   e. None of the above.

10. Inappropriate communication includes:

    a. Frowning.
    b. Eye rolling.
    c. Grimacing.
    d. All of the above.
    e. None of the above.

Matching

The following statements should be matched with the type of response they represent.

A. Judgmental response

B. Advice-giving response

C. Quizzing response

D. Placating response

_____ 1. "Oh, you shouldn't worry so much about the length of time. Just shop around for a while until it is ready, and try not to get yourself so worked up."

_____ 2. "You need to talk to the other patients who are waiting here. They will tell you that we know more about medicine and the prescription-filling process than you do."

_____ 3. "Think back to when you have picked up medication at other pharmacies. I don't believe that you have gotten it as quickly as we are going to give it to you."

_____ 4. "You seem to be the only one concerned about our ability to provide you with the correct medication quickly. All our other patients really love us and don't seem to care about the wait."

_____ 5. "This medication is really not that expensive. I have seen much higher costs."

_____ 6. "You think this is expensive? Have you priced the cost of college lately?"

_____ 7. "If you really think about it, most Americans waste more money in 1 month than the cost of this medication."

_____ 8. "You really have no right to question our prices. I am sure that have had to make a living too."

True or False

_____ 1. Effective communication strategies can help to prevent medication errors and improve the quality of patient care.

_____ 2. Body movements or mannerisms can indicate one's feelings or psychological state of mind.

_____ 3. One of the most important things to remember about verbal communication is that "once it has been said, it can be taken back" because you can always explain why you said what you said.

_____ 4. When communicating using e-mail, it is acceptable to use all upper case letters because this makes the message clearer.

_____ 5. Aggressive behavior, in which an individual displays an overbearing or intimidating attitude, can result in conflict and create a combative atmosphere and a perception of disrespect.

_____ 6. Open-ended questions are questions that can be answered with a simple "yes" or "no."

_____ 7. Older patients generally have low general and health literacy skills.

_____ 8. Sensitivity to the cultural differences is not necessary because to be fair, everyone should receive the same treatment.

_____ 9. There is no excuse for patients to be hostile.

_____ 10. Regardless of outward behaviors, patients need to feel that care and understanding is being extended to them.

Fill in the Blank

1. The statement, "You seem to be the only one concerned about our ability to provide you with the correct medication quickly. All our other patients really love us and don't seem to care about the wait," is considered a _____ response.

2. "Do you have any allergies to medications?" is considered a _____-ended question.

3. The federal law that prohibits the disclosure of protected health information (PHI) to anyone without the patient's permission or outside of the process of providing patient care is called _____.

4. When individuals collaborate or cooperate to accomplish a common goal, they are demonstrating _____.

5. The ability of an individual to read and understand health care information is referred to as _____ _____ skills.

6. _____ patients are the fastest growing population group and account for the highest percentage of medication use (both prescription and over-the-counter).

7. The responsible provision of drug therapy for the purpose of achieving definite outcomes that improve a patient's quality of life is referred to as _____ care.

8. Rolling your eyes is a form of _____ communication.

9. When one displays _____, in which an individual is able to identify with and understand another individual's feelings or difficulties, a caring and trusting relationship may be established.

10. An important part of communication is _____, where a technician can observe any nonverbal communication, better understand the patient's perceptions, and sense the patient's emotions.

Short Answer

1. Describe a situation in a pharmacy where a pharmacy technician would interact with a patient. In this patient encounter scenario, compare and contrast effective and ineffective communication skills using your knowledge of all forms of communication (e.g., verbal and nonverbal).

2. Discuss the use of open-ended questions and close-ended questions. Is one method better than another? Why or why not?

3. Discuss the four types of responses that should be avoided and how these responses might be perceived negatively by the patient, producing an undesirable outcome.

4. Explain the various strategies that can be used by technicians in the pharmacy to identify individuals who lack general and health literacy skills.

5. Teamwork is important in pharmacy. What are the important behaviors that technicians should demonstrate in order to be effective team members?

Word Search

```
S D N E E S O L C B O D Y L A N G U I U V R D O Z
A S S E R T I V I E E M G E Q G A D E R A Y E M T
I N R A U G N A L Y D O B G G U M N I N D I D R G
R V M R A T I S O P T E D A D N Z R V E N L N E H
B D I A G G E S S I V E C U D A I Z S G C A E E S
S A E S T C R A M A U M R G O T P G I O T O O C S
G A U E S B T B M N E N I N M G L C D N E N S G E
R T P G V A O L V W T A R A E B A E S U G A U N T
A A A J N I P D A E O A E L C R A E A E J A L I E
C E C U Q A T E Y T A R A Y E E T D O E I G C T S
A N U S U V L R K L F E K D I V I O W M A E T A I
V G T T I L C Y E I A N S O R N N E M C N I A C A
E E E I Z E G N D S C N D B L O G D L N G M G A E
S E H F Z P H U G O S Z G A N N D W U E A Y O L R
I E T B I P A S S S B A B U N D L A B R E V I P T
S N U L N Q D P A R L R O E E T E G C L R E T Z E
K D P D G M S N U O A C L O S E E N D E D E A J G
T E M E S N E A E V N I O T A C I N U M M O C R N
M C I L A B R E V N O N A J A C O E Y E G I I G I
I E T A E M W O R K E J E E U I J R O N M P N R N
P E A R M G S B G G S P N W T S R I I B D N U E E
D L E T S D D A R A G C O A L O T G U L V N M A D
E C A E M P A T H E T I C E D E U I E H S U M Y E
E V A C C L A N V E I I E N V J I C F T A U O E A
V T N H A S E N D A N J E I N V E E R I L T C V S
I L N I C T H E I U I S S L R E D N E S E U R D E
S G Z C Y H O A M J U S T I F I E T C V B D E A E
S R H C E S O M D N A O G A G O D U E L H G V M H
E L E Y G C O E P P N E C E G T R I I A E I U J A
R N O F O C E E R E M M E E C G I D V P I Y E U M
G R J U S T I F E D I G E A H V R W E I S W C D I
G L R B O D Y A N G U A G E I T E E R E E E A G T
A H E A L T H L I T E R A C Y G A O S I U R R S C
O T T I N A S N O N V E R B O L C P G S G G E E E
I B E T N I D E D N E N E P O I O V M N I L P S E
L R N I V E R B A A I E E H R L A R E E A V N G Z
N T T N L G N I M I N N P S E M E I R F N E A N R
```

AGGRESSIVE

ASSERTIVE

BODYLANGUAGE

CLOSEENDED

COMMUNICATION

EMPATHETIC

HEALTHLITERACY

JUDGING

JUSTIFIED

NONVERBAL

OPENENDED

PASSIVE

PLACATING

QUIZZING

RECEIVER

SENDER

TEAMWORK

VERBAL

Chapter 9

The Human Body: Structure and Function

Learning Outcomes

This chapter reinforces the following learning outcomes discussed in Chapter 9/ The Human Body: Structure and Function of the *Manual for Pharmacy Technicians, 4th edition.*

- Identify the major structures of each of the body systems presented.
- Describe the major functions of each of the body systems presented.
- Describe common diseases and disorders that can develop when something goes wrong in a body system.
- Recognize the role of drug therapy in the common diseases and disorders of the body systems.

Multiple Choice 48

Matching 49

True or False 50

Fill in the Blank 51

Short Answer 52

Crossword Puzzle 53

Multiple Choice

1. The outermost layer of the kidney is called the:

    a. Medulla.
    b. Renal pelvis.
    c. Cortex.
    d. Nephron.

2. The two major parts to the nervous system are the:

    a. Central nervous system and the peripheral nervous system.
    b. Afferent system and the efferent system.
    c. Sympathetic system and the parasympathetic system.
    d. Skeletal muscle and the smooth muscle.

3. When the normal physiological function of a body system becomes abnormal and a disease state occurs, this is known as:

    a. Physiology.
    b. Anatomy.
    c. Pathophysiology.
    d. Abnormal psychology.

4. All of the following are diseases of the nervous system except:

    a. Seizure disorders.
    b. Anxiety disorders.
    c. Hypertension.
    d. Myasthenia gravis.

5. The cardiovascular system is comprised of the:

    a. Heart, lymphatic system, and blood vessels.
    b. Heart, blood vessels, and blood.
    c. Heart, spinal cord, and lymphatic system.
    d. Heart, autonomic nervous system, and kidneys.

6. The right and left sides of the heart are separated into two functional pumps, which do the following:

    a. The right atria and the left ventricle pump blood into the lungs.
    b. The right atria and the right ventricle pump blood into the lungs.
    c. The left atria and left ventricle pump blood into the lungs.
    d. The left atria and the right ventricle pump blood into the lungs.

7. The heart also has a conduction system of nerve pathways that respond to messages from the:

    a. Somatic nervous system.
    b. Afferent division.
    c. Peripheral nervous system.
    d. Autonomic nervous system.

8. This disease is caused when the blood vessels that supply the heart with oxygen become narrowed as the result of atherosclerosis, caused by fatty deposits (plaque) in the inside of blood vessels.

    a. Venous thromboembolism.
    b. Hypertension.
    c. Coronary artery disease.
    d. Heart failure.

9. Stroke, also known as cerebrovascular accidents (CVAs), occur when there is an acute decrease or stoppage of blood flow to a part of the brain, caused by:

    a. A blood clot.
    b. A ruptured blood vessel.
    c. Both a and b.
    d. None of the above.

10. The respiratory system is responsible for gas exchange, which:

    a. Allows oxygen to be taken to cells in the body and carbon dioxide to be removed from the same cells.
    b. Allows carbon dioxide to be taken to cells in the body and oxygen to be removed from the same cells.
    c. Occurs at two levels: at the lungs between the alveoli and the bronchi, and at the cellular level between blood and the tissues.
    d. Occurs at two levels: at the lungs between the trachea and the blood, and at the cellular level between blood and the tissues.

11. The skeleton is made up of _____ bones, each of which varies in size and shape.

    a. 106
    b. 206
    c. 306
    d. 606

12. _____ muscle is the primary muscle found in the internal organs of the body: stomach, intestines, glands, and blood vessels.

   a. Skeletal
   b. Smooth
   c. Sarcolemma
   d. Myofibril

13. Risk factors for osteoporosis include:

   a. Being female (especially after menopause).
   b. A family history of osteoporosis or broken bones.
   c. Cushing's syndrome.
   d. All of the above.
   e. None of the above.

14. The endocrine system works to do all of the following except:

   a. Maintain the body's normal internal balance (homeostasis).
   b. Regulate growth and development.
   c. Produce, use, and store energy.
   d. Control the tear glands around the eye that produce tears to lubricate the eye.

15. The eyes are enclosed by three layers. The outermost layer is the:

   a. Sclera/cornea.
   b. Vitreous humor.
   c. Choroid/ciliary body/iris.
   d. Retina.

16. The part of the ear, which detects changes in position and movement of the head and is responsible for maintaining balance and equilibrium, is called the:

   a. Tympanic membrane.
   b. Organ of Corti.
   c. Auditory canal.
   d. Vestibular apparatus.

17. Treatment for eczema includes all of the following except:

   a. Topical anti-inflammatory creams.
   b. Lubricants.
   c. Antihistamines.
   d. Antiseptics.

18. The skin is a layered structure composed of two layers called:

   a. Keratin and melanin.
   b. Epidermis and dermis.
   c. Sebaceous glands and sweat glands.
   d. Protective pigment and pressure receptors.

19. The female hormones, which are responsible for the development of secondary sex characteristics when an individual reaches puberty, are:

   a. Estrogen and testosterone.
   b. Progesterone and cortisone.
   c. Estrogen and dihydrotesterone.
   d. Estrogen and progesterone.

20. A common cause of erectile dysfunction is:

   a. Diabetes.
   b. Medication.
   c. Atherosclerosis.
   d. All of the above.

Matching

Matching I

Imbalances of the following neurotransmitters are associated with which of the diseases listed below?

A. GABA and acetylcholine

B. dopamine and acetylcholine

C. acetylcholine

D. serotonin and norepinephrine

E. dopamine

F. norepinephrine and dopamine

_____ 1. Alzheimer's disease

_____ 2. Attention deficit hyperactivity disorder

_____ 3. Mood disorders

_____ 4. Parkinson's disease

_____ 5. Psychotic disorders

_____ 6. Seizure disorders

Matching II

Match the following terms with the correct definitions.

A. autoimmunity

B. diastole

C. digestion

D. endocrine

E. endocrine glands

F. gonads

G. pathophysiology

H. peristalsis

I. physiology

J. tolerance

_____ 1. A state of unresponsiveness to a specific antigen or group of antigens to which a person is normally responsive.

_____ 2. The internal secretion of substances into the systemic circulation (bloodstream).

_____ 3. Reproductive organs—testes in the male and ovaries in the female.

_____ 4. Unhealthy function in an individual body system or an organ due to a disease.

_____ 5. A misdirected immune response that happens when the body attacks itself.

_____ 6. Waves of involuntary muscular contractions in the digestive tract.

_____ 7. The study of how living organisms function normally, including such processes as nutrition, movement, and reproduction.

_____ 8. Glands that have no ducts; their secretions are absorbed directly into the blood.

_____ 9. When the heart muscle is relaxed and the chambers are filling with blood; the pressure is at the lowest point in a normal heart.

_____ 10. The process whereby ingested food is broken up into smaller molecules by chemical or mechanical means.

True or False

_____ 1. The ability of the central and peripheral nervous systems to communicate with and regulate the function of organs in the body is possible through the release of neurotransmitters.

_____ 2. Alzheimer's disease is a condition where the myelin sheath is broken down, causing lesions on the nerves, problems with speech, difficulty swallowing, and muscle weakness.

_____ 3. The two most common mood disorders are anxiety and psychosis.

_____ 4. Acute pain typically lasts for months to years and may be accompanied by other symptoms such as sleep problems, lack of appetite, and depression.

_____ 5. Common symptoms of schizophrenia include hallucinations (hearing or seeing things that are not real) and delusions (fixed beliefs that are false).

_____ 6. The white blood cells (leukocytes) are responsible for transporting oxygen to, and carbon dioxide away, from the cells of body tissues.

_____ 7. Two upper chambers are called the ventricles, which are found on the left and right sides of the heart; below them are the two atria.

_____ 8. Veins deliver blood to the heart, and arteries take blood away from the heart.

_____ 9. When the electrical activity of the heart is abnormal, a condition known as anemia develops.

_____ 10. The cause of a stroke can be a blood clot or a blood vessel that has ruptured.

_____ 11. Hypertension is a condition where a person is unable to cope with stressful events.

_____ 12. Skeletal muscle is the primary muscle found in the internal organs of the body: stomach, intestines, glands, and blood vessels.

_____ 13. Osteoarthritis is an inflammatory disease of the joints believed to be an autoimmune disease whereby the body produces specific proteins called antibodies that cause inflammation of a special membrane around the joints.

_____ 14. Generally, problems within the endocrine system are due to one of two things: either too little or too much of a hormone is produced.

_____ 15. The organs of the immune system are connected with one another and with other organs of the body by a network of lymphatic vessels similar to blood vessels.

_____ 16. The ultimate goal of inflammation is to bring more help from the immune system to destroy the invaders, remove the dead cells, and begin the process of tissue healing and repair.

_____ 17. Drugs called antiarrhythmias are commonly used to treat and prevent allergies.

_____ 18. The pulmonary system terminates in single-layered cell structures called bronchioles, where the exchange of gases takes place between the lungs and the blood.

_____ 19. Chronic Obstructive Pulmonary Disease (COPD) includes two conditions known as emphysema and chronic obstructive bronchitis.

_____ 20. Actin and myosin are responsible for making a muscle contract and relax.

_____ 21. An individual suffering from hyperthyroidism can be treated with thyroid hormone replacement.

_____ 22. Diabetes insipidus is treated with insulin.

Fill in the Blank

1. _____ is the study of body structure.

2. The study of the collective functions and processes of the body systems is known as _____.

3. Within the peripheral nervous system, the _____ division brings information such as temperature from the external environment as well as information on the status of internal organs, for example heart rate, to the brain.

4. The _____ nervous system transmits signals to the skeletal muscles of the body, which are under voluntary control.

5. The sympathetic nervous system works when the body is under stress and is best described as that which causes the _____ response.

6. The heart is separated into _____ chambers.

7. _____ is a disease of the lungs characterized by inflammation of the bronchioles, increased mucus secretion, and abnormal contractions of the smooth muscles in the bronchioles, which leads to the narrowing of the airway passages.

8. _____ is a condition that affects the bones, where the structure of the bone changes from a dense and heavy structure to a thinner and lighter one because of a loss of proteins and minerals such as calcium and phosphate.

9. Type _____ diabetes (previously known as juvenile diabetes) is characterized by a lack of insulin production from the pancreas.

10. Type _____ diabetes is the most common type of diabetes, and it is characterized as either decreased production of insulin or an abnormal sensitivity of the tissues to the insulin that is present.

11. The body's complex defense system, called the _____ system, provides constant protection against invasion by foreign substances or organisms.

12. When the outermost layer of the eye and the inner eyelids become inflamed, the condition called _____ occurs, commonly referred to as pink eye. It can be caused by an allergic reaction or infection by a virus or bacteria.

13. _____ _____ occurs when the skin of an individual becomes exposed to an allergen, chemicals, metals, or plants, causing a red rash, blisters, or wheals, as well as itching and burning.

14. The condition of inflammation of the epidermis, causing patches of red, dry, or crusty flaking areas that itch, is called _____.

15. HIV-AIDS, genital herpes, hepatitis C, human papillomavirus [HPV], genital warts, chlamydia, gonorrhea, syphilis, trichomoniasis, and pelvic inflammatory disease are all examples of _____ _____ _____.

16. In some men, especially those greater than 60 years of age, the prostate gland expands so much that it presses against the urethra, causing bladder problems such as frequent urination, a weak stream of urine, and urgency or leaking of urine. This condition is called _____ _____ _____.

Short Answer

1. Describe the functions of the kidneys.

2. Describe the basic anatomy and physiology of the nervous system.

3. Explain how oxygen reaches cells in the human body. What systems are involved?

4. What is the purpose of the immune system; in general terms, how does it work?

5. How is food turned into energy in the human body?

Crossword Puzzle

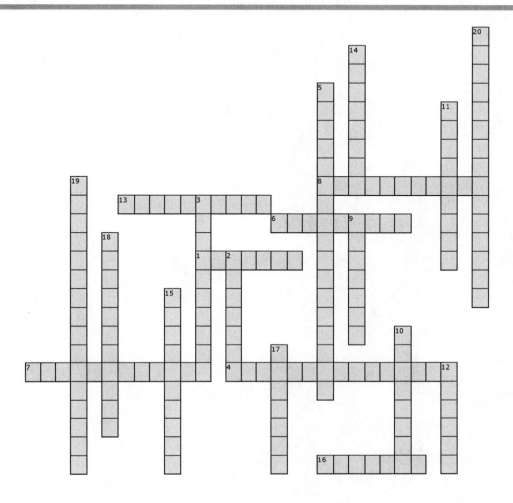

Across:

1. When the heart muscle is contracting
4. Glands that have no ducts
6. A state of unresponsiveness to a specific antigen
7. A misdirected immune response that happens when the body attacks itself
8. Involuntary muscular contractions in the digestive tract
13. The mental process of becoming aware of or recognizing an object or idea
16. A substance that causes production of an antibody

Down:

2. To form and give off
3. The study of how living organisms function normally
5. Disease where myelin sheath is broken down, lesions appear
9. The study of body structure
10. When the heart muscle is relaxed
11. The process whereby ingested food is broken up into smaller molecules
12. Cardiovascular accident
14. A structure of a cell that selectively receives and binds a specific substance
15. Disease with tremors
17. Regulates the activity of certain cells
18. Abnormal rhythms
19. An instrument for measuring blood pressure
20. Unhealthy function in an individual body system

Chapter 10

Drug Classifications and Pharmacologic Actions

Learning Outcomes

This chapter reinforces the following learning outcomes discussed in Chapter 10/ Drug Classifications and Pharmacologic Actions of the *Manual for Pharmacy Technicians, 4th edition.*

- Identify the common drug names for each classification.
- Describe the important actions and/or therapeutic uses for the major classes of drugs.
- Describe the most common or most serious adverse effects for the major classes of drugs.
- List special precautions for the major classes of drugs.

Multiple Choice 56

Matching 58

True or False 59

Fill in the Blank 60

Short Answer 61

Alphabet Soup 62

Multiple Choice

1. An ideal drug would have this important characteristic:

   a. Effectiveness for its therapeutic use.
   b. Safety even if large quantities are ingested.
   c. No adverse effects.
   d. All of the above.
   e. None of the above.

2. Drugs can be classified by:

   a. Medical conditions.
   b. Body organ systems.
   c. Type of action.
   d. All of the above.
   e. None of the above.

3. Antiepileptic drugs may be used for:

   a. Migraine prevention.
   b. Psychiatric disorders.
   c. Painful facial nerve condition called trigeminal neuralgia.
   d. All of the above.
   e. None of the above.

4. An FDA-approved Medication Guide must be dispensed with all prescriptions for antiepileptic drugs to warn patients about the potential risk of:

   a. Liver toxicity.
   b. Suicidal thoughts or behavior.
   c. Weight gain.
   d. All of the above.
   e. None of the above.

5. The goal for treatment of Parkinson's disease (PD) is to:

   a. Cure the disease.
   b. Keep the disease from spreading.
   c. Maintain function and quality of life.
   d. All of the above.
   e. None of the above.

6. Drug therapy for Parkinson's disease is focused on:

   a. Decreasing acetylcholine and increasing dopamine.
   b. Increasing acetylcholine and decreasing dopamine.
   c. Increasing acetylcholine and increasing dopamine.
   d. Decreasing acetylcholine and decreasing dopamine.

7. Alzheimer's disease signs and symptoms include:

   a. Uncontrollable tremors.
   b. High fever and rash.
   c. Memory impairment and behavioral changes.
   d. Muscle spasms and weakness.

8. Which of the following statements about multiple sclerosis (MS) is *not* true?

   a. It is a progressive neurological disorder affecting the brain and the spinal cord.
   b. Its onset is generally between the ages of 18 and 45 and often affects women more than men.
   c. In MS, the myelin sheath that covers neurons degenerates, causing a disruption of nerve transmission.
   d. Symptoms may include memory loss and confusion.

9. Goals of headache therapy include all of the following except:

   a. Ability to maintain normal activities.
   b. Provide quick relief of headache pain.
   c. Reduce frequency of attacks.
   d. Maximize the amount of medications needed.

10. Neuropathic pain may be due to:

    a. The persistent stimulation of nerve fibers.
    b. Nerve damage in the central or peripheral nervous system.
    c. All of the above.
    d. None of the above.

11. The drugs used in the treatment of the mood disorders work by altering the various chemicals, called neurotransmitters, found at the nerve junctions in the brain, which include:

    a. Norepinephrine and epinephrine.
    b. Serotonin and dopamine.
    c. All of the above.
    d. None of the above.

12. First-line therapy of ADHD is:

    a. Atomoxetine (Strattera).
    b. Bupropion (Wellbutrin).
    c. Venlafaxine (Effexor).
    d. All of the above.
    e. None of the above.

13. The goal of treatment for cholesterol and triglycerides is to:

    a. Reduce low density lipoprotein (LDL) levels and reduce high density lipoprotein (HDL) levels.
    b. Reduce low density lipoprotein (LDL) levels and increase high density lipoprotein (HDL) levels.
    c. Increase low density lipoprotein (LDL) levels and increase high density lipoprotein (HDL) levels.
    d. Increase low density lipoprotein (LDL) levels and reduce high density lipoprotein (HDL) levels.

14. Which of the following is *not* true about diuretics?

    a. Thiazide diuretics are well tolerated by patients.
    b. Blood glucose control in patients with diabetes may be altered by thiazide diuretics.
    c. Patients who are taking thiazide diuretics may be more sensitive to sun.
    d. All of the above.
    e. None of the above.

15. Which is *not* true about angiotensin-converting enzyme inhibitors (ACE inhibitors)?

    a. ACE inhibitors may slow or prevent the development of kidney disease in diabetic patients.
    b. ACE inhibitors may increase survival, alleviate symptoms, and decrease hospitalization in patients with heart failure.
    c. The ACE inhibitors have a –pril ending on the name.
    d. ACE inhibitors can clear up bothersome dry coughs.

16. Calcium channel blockers are used for:

    a. Chest pain (angina pectoris).
    b. Heart rhythm disturbances.
    c. Migraine headache.
    d. All of the above.
    e. None of the above.

17. An important consideration in choosing dosage regimens for nitrates is:

    a. The development of tolerance.
    b. That after 24 hours of continuous therapy, nitrates no longer work.
    c. That increasing the dose does not restore efficacy.
    d. All of the above.
    e. None of the above.

18. Which of the following medications is not a type of bronchodilators?

    a. Beta2-agonists.
    b. Acetylcholine blockers.
    c. Anticholinergics.
    d. Methylxanthines.

19. Inhaled corticosteroids are:

    a. Avoided in children due to reports that they affect growth.
    b. Known to cause thrush (fungus of the throat and mouth) in some patients.
    c. Safe for long-term treatment of asthma.
    d. Avoided in patients with COPD.

20. Expectorants are controversial because:

    a. There is little scientific evidence to show that they effectively aid in expectoration.
    b. They require a prescription.
    c. They are very expensive.
    d. They may not be used in combination with other medications.

21. Nonsteroidal anti-inflammatory drugs (NSAIDs):

    a. Have analgesic (pain-relieving) properties.
    b. Have antipyretic (fever-reducing) properties.
    c. Can cause serious bleeding and ulcers in the stomach.
    d. All of the above.
    e. None of the above.

22. The best medications used to treat muscle pain and spasm are:

    a. Cyclobenzaprine (Flexeril).
    b. Diazepam (Valium).
    c. Tizanidine (Zanaflex).
    d. None of the above.

23. Due to the subjective nature of pain, the standard assessment of pain is determined:

    a. By the patient's facial expressions.
    b. By speaking to the patient's spouse or caregiver.
    c. Using pain scales.
    d. None of the above.

24. Insulin:

    a.   Is the mainstay of treatment for many patients with diabetes insipidus.

    b.   Can be given only by subcutaneous or intravenous injection.

    c.   Requires a prescription.

    d.   Varieties all have the same onset of action, but may differ in the length of time (after the injection) that the effects last.

25. The following is an antithyroid drug:

    a.   Propylthiouracil (PTU).

    b.   Levothyroxine (Synthroid).

    c.   All of the above.

    d.   None of the above.

26. Which of the following statements about antihistamines is *not* true?

    a.   Antihistamines reduce or prevent symptoms of allergic rhinitis.

    b.   Antihistamines are often included in cold products because of their drying effects on mucosal secretions.

    c.   Antihistamines have been shown to effectively shorten the duration of the common cold.

    d.   All of the above are *not* true.

    e.   None of the above is *not* true.

27. Intranasal corticosteroids are:

    a.   Used for rhinitis and other allergic or inflammatory conditions of the nose.

    b.   Very effective agents due to immediate benefit.

    c.   Used frequently during the day due to short duration of action.

    d.   All of the above.

    e.   None of the above.

28. The histamine-2 receptor antagonists (H2 antagonists):

    a.   Are the same as the proton pump inhibitors.

    b.   Block the same histamine receptor than the antihistamines used for allergic conditions.

    c.   Are available for the oral route only.

    d.   May be used in drug regimens directed at eradicating *H. pylori*.

29. Agents to treat inflammatory bowel disease (IBD) include:

    a.   Aminosalicylates.

    b.   Immunosuppressive agents.

    c.   Monoclonal antibodies.

    d.   All of the above.

    e.   None of the above.

30. A common ophthalmic disease is:

    a.   Conjunctivitis.

    b.   Glaucoma.

    c.   Dryness of the eyes.

    d.   All of the above.

    e.   None of the above.

Matching

Match the following vitamins with their synonyms:

A. Vitamin A

B. Vitamin E

C. Vitamin B_1

D. Vitamin B_2

E. Vitamin B_5

F. Vitamin B_6

G. Vitamin B_{12}

H. Vitamin B_3

_____ 1. Cyanocobalamin

_____ 2. Niacin (Nicotinic Acid)

_____ 3. Pantothenic Acid

_____ 4. Pyridoxine

_____ 5. Retinol

_____ 6. Riboflavin

_____ 7. Thiamine

_____ 8. Tocopherol

True or False

_____ 1. Antiepileptic agents should not be discontinued abruptly.

_____ 2. There may be differences in the bioavailability (extent of absorption) of the antiepileptic generics versus brand-name drugs, which may correlate to an increase in adverse effects/ toxicities or an increase in seizure frequency.

_____ 3. Phenytoin is an injectable medication that is converted to fosphenytoin (Cerebyx) in the body.

_____ 4. Phenytoin IV must only be mixed in dextrose. If phenytoin is mixed with normal saline, a precipitate will form.

_____ 5. The most common agents used in MS patients are those to prevent relapses and disease progression, and they have become known as the ABC therapy (Avonex, Betaseron, Copaxone).

_____ 6. The most common class of medications used for the treatment of migraines is Interferon-β-1b (Betaseron).

_____ 7. Antidepressant medications are often used in the treatment of neuropathic pain.

_____ 8. The drugs used in the treatment of mood disorders work by altering the various chemicals, called neurotransmitters, found at the nerve junctions in the brain and include norepinephrine, epinephrine, serotonin, and dopamine.

_____ 9. Monoamine oxidase inhibitors (MAO-Is) are thought to be effective and safe antidepressants because they have few drug or food interactions.

_____ 10. Drugs used for anxiety (anxiolytics) include SSRIs, benzodiazepines, SNRIs, TCAs, and buspirone (Buspar).

_____ 11. Psychosis is a mental disorder in which a person's capacity to recognize reality is distorted.

_____ 12. Benzodiazepines may and should be stopped abruptly at 6 months because they are habit forming.

_____ 13. The atypical antipsychotic agents have been shown to be more effective than the older agents.

_____ 14. Omega-3 fatty acids (Lovaza), commonly found in fish oil, have been shown to reduce triglyceride levels in patients with very high triglycerides in their blood (hypertriglyceridemia).

_____ 15. The HMG-CoA reductase inhibitors are also known as "statins."

_____ 16. Loop diuretics are less potent diuretics and have fewer effects on electrolytes such as sodium, potassium, chloride, calcium, and magnesium than the thiazides.

_____ 17. ACE inhibitors may slow or prevent the development of kidney disease in diabetic patients and increase survival, alleviate symptoms, and decrease hospitalization in patients with heart failure.

_____ 18. The ACE inhibitors have a –olol ending on the name.

_____ 19. After 24 hours of continuous therapy, nitrates no longer work.

_____ 20. Asthma inhalers are meant to treat an acute attack (i.e., "quick-relief").

_____ 21. Patients with hypertension, heart disease, overactive thyroid, diabetes mellitus, or an enlarged prostate gland should use caution if taking decongestants.

_____ 22. Adequate calcium intake is essential for the prevention and treatment of osteoporosis.

_____ 23. All NSAIDs can cause serious bleeding and ulcers in the stomach.

_____ 24. All muscle relaxants cause sedation.

_____ 25. Opioid analgesics control pain, reduce inflammation, lower fever, and suppress cough and diarrhea.

_____ 26. Insulin can be given only by subcutaneous or intravenous injection.

_____ 27. Oral hypoglycemic agents are used to lower blood sugar in Type 1 diabetes.

_____ 28. Diseases of the thyroid gland include hypothyroidism (underproduction of thyroid hormone) and hyperthyroidism (overproduction of thyroid hormone).

_____ 29. Antihistamines often cause excitation, but a paradoxical reaction of drowsiness rather than excitation is sometimes seen in children and the elderly.

_____ 30. Since the antacid aluminum hydroxide commonly causes constipation and the antacid magnesium hydroxide commonly causes diarrhea, these antacids are combined to try to avoid either constipation or diarrhea.

_____ 31. When treating nausea and vomiting, OTC medications are generally used first before moving to prescription medications.

_____ 32. Inflammatory bowel disease is usually controlled by the use of a single agent.

_____ 33. Diseases on or near the surface of the eye are most often treated with oral topical medications.

_____ 34. Eye drops may have systemic effects.

_____ 35. Ophthalmic vasoconstrictors, or "decongestants," are commonly used to reduce redness in the eyes from minor irritations, are available over the counter for this purpose, and may be used indefinitely.

_____ 36. Topical ear treatments are commonly used for conditions involving the middle or inner ear.

_____ 37. Oral contraceptives are used to prevent pregnancy, to regulate menstruation, to treat endometriosis, to treat polycystic ovary syndrome, and to treat acne vulgaris.

_____ 38. A woman is considered to have infertility problems after attempting to conceive for over 3 years without success.

_____ 39. Benign prostatic hypertrophy (BPH) is a non-cancerous enlargement of the prostate gland that develops in older men and women.

_____ 40. The severity, site, and source of infection; characteristics of the antibiotic; and characteristics of the patient are all considered when an antibiotic is selected.

_____ 41. Penicillin allergies are estimated to occur in 5 to 8% of the population and can be fatal.

_____ 42. Patients who are allergic to penicillin should not take the macrolides.

_____ 43. Fluoroquinolones may be used in the general population for treatment of urinary tract infections, respiratory infections, and gastrointestinal infections and as single-dose therapy for some sexually transmitted diseases.

_____ 44. Vancomycin is usually given intravenously or orally for treatment of systemic infections.

_____ 45. The Centers for Disease Control and Prevention, an agency of the U.S. Government, has published guidelines for the prevention and treatment of TB.

_____ 46. Herpes simplex virus causes the very painful symptoms of shingles and the potentially serious cases of chicken pox in people with weakened immune systems (e.g., children with leukemia).

_____ 47. Anti-HIV antivirals have been developed that may be effectively used as monotherapy.

_____ 48. Liposomal amphotericin B formulations are less toxic to the kidneys and cause fewer infusion-related adverse events when compared with conventional amphotericin.

_____ 49. Colony-stimulating factors are used to increase red blood cells.

_____ 50. Because anticoagulants slow clot formation, the main concern with anticoagulant therapy is excessive bleeding.

Fill in the Blank

1. Antiepileptic agents, also called _____, are used to reduce the frequency of seizures.

2. _____ _____ is a condition of repetitive seizures with little or no interruption between them.

3. The most common class of medications used for the treatment of migraines is the serotonin 5-HT1 receptor agonists, or the _____.

4. _____ pain may be due to the persistent stimulation of nerve fibers or nerve damage in the central or peripheral nervous system.

5. Many medications now contain _____ _____ _____, which are strong warnings that need to be considered carefully prior to prescribing the medication to a patient.

6. _____ antidepressants (TCAs) were the most widely used antidepressants for many years and have the recognizable stem of –triptyline.

7. _____ disorder, also called manic-depressive disorder, is characterized by extreme mood swings.

8. _____ is a mental disorder in which a person's capacity to recognize reality is distorted.

9. _____, or memory loss, is an adverse effect but is desirable when these drugs are used for sedation during painful medical procedures.

10. _____ decrease blood pressure by decreasing the blood volume.

11. _____ are the most commonly used medicines for treating angina pectoris.

12. _____ are commonly used to suppress inflammation and the immune response, which is useful in a wide spectrum of diseases, including asthma, allergic reactions, lupus, ulcerative colitis, psoriasis, rheumatoid arthritis, bursitis, and organ transplantation.

13. _____ is a disease that affects both women and men characterized by a loss of bone, resulting in misshapen bone such as curvature of the backbone seen in the elderly, or in easily broken bones.

14. _____ was one of the first antibiotics developed and can be identified by the –cillin ending on the drug name.

15. Gentamicin, tobramycin, and amikacin belong to the drug class of _____ antibiotics and are able to kill many organisms, including many hospital-acquired organisms.

16. A reaction referred to as Red Man Syndrome may occur if the drug _____ is given too rapidly.

17. _____ _____virus is the cause of fever blisters or cold sores.

18. _____ is the most commonly used oral anticoagulant.

19. Vitamin _____ may be given to reverse the effects of the anticoagulant warfarin.

20. _____ is the primary mineral found inside cells and its imbalance adversely affects cellular metabolism and nerve and muscle function.

Short Answer

1. Identify the common drug names, important actions and/or therapeutic uses, most common or most serious adverse effects, and special precautions for drugs that affect the nervous system.

2. Identify the common drug names, important actions and/or therapeutic uses, most common or most serious adverse effects, and special precautions for drugs that affect the cardiovascular system.

3. Identify the common drug names, important actions and/or therapeutic uses, most common or most serious adverse effects, and special precautions for drugs that affect the respiratory system.

4. Identify the common drug names, important actions and/or therapeutic uses, most common or most serious adverse effects, and special precautions for drugs that affect the musculoskeletal system.

5. Identify the common drug names, important actions and/or therapeutic uses, most common or most serious adverse effects, and special precautions for drugs that affect the endocrine system.

6. Identify the common drug names, important actions and/or therapeutic uses, most common or most serious adverse effects, and special precautions for drugs that affect the immune system.

7. Identify the common drug names, important actions and/or therapeutic uses, most common or most serious adverse effects, and special precautions for drugs that affect the gastrointestinal system.

8. Identify the common drug names, important actions and/or therapeutic uses, most common or most serious adverse effects, and special precautions for drugs that affect the urinary system.

9. Identify the common drug names, important actions and/or therapeutic uses, most common or most serious adverse effects, and special precautions for drugs that are used for eyes, ears, and skin therapy

10. Identify the common drug names, important actions and/or therapeutic uses, most common or most serious adverse effects, and special precautions for drugs that are used as anti-infectives.

11. Identify the common drug names, important actions and/or therapeutic uses, most common or most serious adverse effects, and special precautions for drugs that are used for HIV and cancer treatment.

Part
2

Alphabet Soup

Many acronyms are used in the medical profession. Fill in the full name of each acronym below.

a.   USAN

b.   PD

c.   MS

d.   OTC

e.   SSRIs

f.   SNRIs

g.   MAOIs

h.   TCAs

i.   OCD

j.   IM

k.   EPS

l.   ADHD

m.   LDL

n.   HDL

o.   TG

p.   CAD

q.   ACE inhibitors

r.   ARBs

s.   COPD

t.   MDI

u.   NSAIDs

v.   PTU

w.   MMR

x.   DTaP

y.   HPV

z.   PUD

aa.   GERD

bb.   MOM

cc.   IBD

dd.   SPF

ee.   FSH

ff.   hMG

gg.   HCG

hh.   HRT

ii.   BPH

jj.   ED

kk.   VRE

ll.   TB

mm.   HIV

nn.   RSV

oo.   CMV

pp.   CSF

qq.   EPO

rr.   HIT

ss.   UFH

tt.   LMWHs

uu.   DVT

vv.   AMI

ww.   RDA

xx.   CAM

Chapter 11

Basic Pharmaceutics, Pharmacokinetics, and Pharmacodynamics

Multiple Choice 64

Matching 65

True or False 66

Fill in the Blank 66

Short Answer 66

Word Search 67

Learning Outcomes

This chapter reinforces the following learning outcomes discussed in Chapter 11/ Basic Pharmaceutics, Pharmacokinetics, and Pharmacodynamics of the *Manual for Pharmacy Technicians, 4th edition.*

- Define the study of biopharmaceutics.
- List and describe the four major processes that make up the study of pharmacokinetics.
- Describe factors that can alter the absorption of a medication.
- Describe how medications are distributed within the body, including factors that affect medication distribution in the body.
- List and describe the two most common types of drug interactions.
- Define pharmacodynamics.
- Describe how medications are eliminated from the body, including factors (e.g., disease states) that can increase or decrease elimination of a medication.
- Describe the steps that must occur before a medication can exert its effect on the body.
- Describe potential problems that can occur when a product formulation is disrupted or when absorption, distribution, metabolism, or elimination is altered and how these alterations can affect the pharmacodynamics of a medication.

Multiple Choice

1. Any given tablet will contain not only active drug but also:

   a. Binders.
   b. Fillers.
   c. Preservatives.
   d. All of the above.

2. ADME refers to:

   a. Administration, duration, metabolism, excretion.
   b. Absorption, disintegration, metabolism, excretion.
   c. Absorption, dissolution, metabolism, excretion.
   d. Absorption, distribution, metabolism, excretion.

3. The bioavailability of an agent depends on:

   a. The amount of drug dissolved.
   b. Its dosage form.
   c. Its route of administration.
   d. All of the above.
   e. None of the above.

4. This route of drug administration avoids first-pass metabolism.

   a. Oral.
   b. Inhalation.
   c. All of the above.
   d. None of the above.

5. Examples of medications whose levels are measured in the blood include:

   a. Antiepileptic agents such as phenytoin, carbamazepine, valproic acid, and phenobarbital.
   b. Digoxin.
   c. Gentamicin, tobramycin, and vancomycin.
   d. All of the above.
   e. None of the above.

6. Pharmacokinetics is defined as the study of:

   a. The manufacture of medications for effective delivery into the body.
   b. The movement of a drug through the body.
   c. The relationship between the concentration of a drug in the body and the response or outcome observed or measured in a patient.
   d. Pharmacy products' molecular structures.

7. Medications given intravenously are administered directly into the vein; therefore:

   a. Are 100% bioavailable.
   b. Are dosed the same as medications given orally.
   c. May have an intravenous dose that is much higher than doses given orally.
   d. Are subject to first-pass metabolism.

8. Metabolism:

   a. Occurs in the liver.
   b. Occurs in the small intestines.
   c. Produces metabolites.
   d. All of the above.
   e. None of the above.

9. Metabolites can be:

   a. Inactive.
   b. Toxic.
   c. Active.
   d. All of the above.
   e. None of the above.

10. The most common location of drug excretion in the body is the:

    a. Liver.
    b. Kidneys.
    c. Intestines.
    d. Lungs.

Matching

Match the following terms with the correct definitions below:

A. absorption

B. bioavailability

C. biopharmaceutics

D. clearance

E. cytochrome P450 (CYP)

F. disintegration

G. dissolution

H. drug interaction

I. first-pass metabolism

J. half-life

K. loading dose

L. metabolism

M. metabolite

N. pharmacodynamics

O. pharmacokinetics

P. therapeutic level

Q. volume of distribution

_____ 1. A breakdown product of a medication that has undergone metabolism.

_____ 2. A group of enzymes that metabolize drugs.

_____ 3. A larger first dose given to quickly achieve a high drug concentration in the body.

_____ 4. The process of medication entering the bloodstream or systemic circulation.

_____ 5. The blood level at which most patients receive a medication's desired effect with minimal side effects.

_____ 6. The breakdown of medication from its original solid formulation.

_____ 7. The breakdown of medication in the body.

_____ 8. The dissolving of medication into solution, usually in the stomach and intestinal tract.

_____ 9. The extent of a medication's outreach to various tissues and spaces throughout the body.

_____ 10. The impact of a drug or food product on the amount or activity of another drug in the body.

_____ 11. The metabolism (breaking down) of orally ingested medications by the liver and small intestine before they reach the main bloodstream.

_____ 12. The percentage of an administered dose of a medication that reaches the bloodstream.

_____ 13. The study of the manufacture of medications for effective delivery into the body.

_____ 14. The study of the movement of a drug through the body during the following phases: absorption, distribution, metabolism, and excretion.

_____ 15. The study of the relationship between the concentration of a drug in the body and the response or outcome observed or measured in a patient.

_____ 16. The time that it takes for 50% of a drug to be eliminated from the body.

_____ 17. The total removal of a drug via metabolism and/ or excretion.

True or False

____ 1. Disintegration is the dissolving of medication into solution, usually in the stomach and intestinal tract.

____ 2. Some medications that are administered intravenously are metabolized (broken down) before they reach the main bloodstream, which is referred to as first-pass metabolism.

____ 3. The medication bound to blood proteins is active and exerts its pharmacologic effect while it is bound to the protein.

____ 4. The therapeutic level for medications is the level at which most patients receive the desired effect with minimal side effects.

____ 5. In general, medications with a large volume of distribution will have a higher blood concentration, whereas medications with a small volume of distribution will have a lower blood concentration.

____ 6. If a medication is widely distributed throughout the body and the prescriber wants the medication to start working quickly, sometimes a loading dose of the medication will be given to more quickly achieve a higher drug concentration in the body.

____ 7. Most medications require a loading dose.

____ 8. Most drug metabolism occurs in the kidneys, although significant metabolism can occur in the small intestine.

____ 9. The most common enzymes that metabolize drugs belong to a family of enzymes called the cytochrome P450 (CYP) system.

____ 10. A "pro-drug" is where a drug is administered in an inactive form, which is metabolized or converted to the active component.

Fill in the Blank

1. _____ is the study of the manufacture of medications for effective delivery into the body.

2. In pharmacokinetics, _____ refers to the amount of medication that enters the bloodstream or systemic circulation.

3. _____ is the dissolving of medication into solution.

4. The term _____ refers to the percentage of an administered dose of a medication that reaches the bloodstream.

5. _____ is the main protein that binds medications in the blood.

6. In pharmacokinetics, the _____ of medication is the breakdown of medication in the body.

7. _____ refers to the irreversible removal of a drug or metabolite from a body fluid.

8. A _____ _____ is defined as the impact of a drug on the amount or activity of another drug in the body.

9. The most common way to detect the presence of kidney disease is to measure blood levels of _____, a substance that is normally produced in muscles and is cleared from the body by the kidneys.

10. Medications that augment or enhance a signal normally communicated in a cell are called _____.

11. The time that it takes for 50% of a drug to be eliminated from the body is called the _____.

Short Answer

1. Explain why the pharmacy technician who prepares prescriptions for dispensing should have a basic understanding of biopharmaceutics, pharmacokinetics, and pharmacodynamics.

2. List and describe the four major processes that make up the study of pharmacokinetics.

3. List and describe the two most common types of drug interactions.

4. Define pharmacodynamics.

5. Describe the steps that must occur before a medication can exert its effect on the body.

Word Search

```
M Y T I C H Y T I L I B A L A I V A O B E C O S I
I T N F T L E D I S I N T I G R A T I O N U I S N
T T O E N B I O P H A R M A C E U T I C S I S E C
S C I M A N Y D O C A M R A H P T D S O S C E L U
N N T P H A R M A C O D Y N A M M E R C U T A I L
A S A T T I I L T A T N N I A A F N I L C C M M I
L A N T A I I G F E O O O R I O M C S N A S I O
N N I A I I X O L I I A E I L I A O O A A O I N F
A T M R T I U R D T A F A F T Y S B M N R O L N L
R T I A R I T L C S I M L P D E Y I A I A I O A T
A F L E T E I I S F G A O O S M R F M N E S B T A
E O E I R T R A L S H S C T V O S C I A L O A I T
L I E C L O P A B L B A A E B E C I X L C D T O S
C R X O T H G D A M S I N E M S A A E F E U N T
A E R N S O N T T R N O I T C A R E T N I L M R B
A I A R S I H M A S C I T E N I K O C A M R A H P
Y V I S D B C H E L E V E L C I T U E P A R E H T
I F A A N I P A S A N A D I S S O L U T I Y A A C
I E O A B O B B E E O T I O U I Y T C T E R A L R O
L L M B I P I T C H I C Y T O C H R E T I P T S O
I B L S O H O N M E T I L O A T E M I T T I S C A
B N O C P A A I O S A A V I B G O L O S O T T I F
A N A I H R V I D A R M H O M D O Y R D N E T L S
L P D T A M A E N X G N M I S B S I T O N N O T M
I S A E R A I C I T E E H M A P F U E S S A O E B
A U L N M C L N R E T V I T C H F T D E C C V F I
V C I I A E A A O C N A E G A M E T A B O L I S M
A R L K C U B R L H I M M U B L A O D O N G S N L
O M I O E T I E C I S C I R I N T E R A C T I O O
I C E C U I L A A I I S O D H A L V I E N K V A N
B E O A T I I L E N D A E X R E T O I N A T R A T
V A N M R I E C H I M C Y T O C H R O M E A I R C
D B I R A B S O R P T I O N N N I I L O B A T E M
B O P E S S I E A D I S S O L U T E O N P I H D P
C S I H D I S S O L U T I O N I M E X C R E T I O
B T L P A L B L N I A P E N O N L E O S M C U U O
```

ABSORPTION
BIOAVAILABILITY
BIOPHARMACEUTICS
CLEARANCE
CYTOCHROME
DISINTEGRATION
DISSOLUTION
DOSE
DRUG
ELIMINATION

EXCRETION
FIRSTPASS
HALFLIFE
INTERACTION
LOADING
METABOLISM
METABOLITE
PHARMACODYNAMICS
PHARMACOKINETICS
THERAPEUTICLEVEL

Chapter 12

Medication Dosage Forms and Routes of Administration

Learning Outcomes

This chapter reinforces the following learning outcomes discussed in Chapter 12/ Medication Dosage Forms and Routes of Administration of the *Manual for Pharmacy Technicians, 4th edition.*

- Explain why medications are often available in more than one dosage form.
- List three advantages of liquid medication dosage forms over other dosage forms.
- List three disadvantages of solid medication dosage forms.
- Outline characteristics of solutions, emulsions, and suspensions.
- Describe two situations in which an ointment may be preferred over a cream.
- Explain the differences in use among various solid medication dosage forms such as tablets, capsules, lozenges, powders, and granules.
- List six routes of administration by which drugs may enter or be applied to the body.
- Identify special considerations for five routes of administration.
- List five parenteral routes of administration.
- Distinguish between sublingual and buccal routes.

Multiple Choice 70

Matching 71

True or False 71

Fill in the Blank 72

Short Answer 72

Alphabet Soup 72

Crossword Puzzle 73

Multiple Choice

1. Common medication vehicles are:

   a. Water, alcohol, glycerin, and mineral oil.
   b. Jars, bottles, and vials.
   c. Tablets, capsules, and caplets.
   d. Fillers, binders, and dispersants.

2. The advantage of syrups is that:

   a. Their sweet taste can disguise the unpleasant taste of medications.
   b. Only a portion of the medication dissolved in the syrup comes in contact with the taste buds.
   c. The thick nature of syrups also has a soothing effect on irritated tissues of the throat.
   d. All of the above.
   e. None of the above.

3. Irrigants are used to wash or cleanse part of the body such as:

   a. The eyes.
   b. The urinary bladder.
   c. Open wounds.
   d. All of the above.
   e. None of the above.

4. Patients should be warned about alcohol content of elixirs because:

   a. Alcohol can have undesired interactions with other medications the patients may be taking.
   b. Medication may not completely dissolve in alcohol.
   c. Alcohol may alter flavor of medication.
   d. All of the above.
   e. None of the above.

5. Glycerin may be used in:

   a. Oral medications.
   b. Otic medications.
   c. Ophthalmic medications.
   d. All of the above.
   e. None of the above.

6. Solid medication dosage forms allow for delivery of medications:

   a. Orally.
   b. Rectally.
   c. Vaginally.
   d. All of the above.
   e. None of the above.

7. Reasons for enteric coating of tablets include:

   a. To improve flavor.
   b. To protect the lining of the intestines from irritation by the drug.
   c. All of the above.
   d. None of the above.

8. Administration methods of various medications in hard gelatin capsules include:

   a. Swallowing whole.
   b. Opening and sprinkling the powdered ingredients inside on food or in water before taking.
   c. Inhaling through the mouth into the lungs using a mechanical device that punctures the capsule and releases the powder.
   d. All of the above.
   e. None of the above.

9. Caplets are also known as:

   a. Troches.
   b. Pastilles.
   c. Lozenges.
   d. All of the above.
   e. None of the above.

10. Creams may be preferred over ointments because:

    a. They are easier to spread.
    b. They have a cooling effect on the skin.
    c. In the case of O/W creams, they are easier to wash off with water.
    d. All of the above.
    e. None of the above.

Matching

Match the following terms with the correct definitions.

A. Oral

B. Buccal

C. Sublingual

D. Subgingival

E. Enteral

F. Parenteral

G. Intra-arterial

H. Intra-articular

I. Intracardiac

J. Intradermal

K. Intrathecal

L. Intravenous

M. Intraventricular

N. Intravesicular

O. Intravitreal

P. Subcutaneous

Q. Intranasal

R. Ophthalmic

S. Otic

T. Percutaneous

U. Rectal

V. Topical

W. Transdermal

_____ 1. Applied to skin or mucous membranes

_____ 2. By way of the intestine

_____ 3. Bypassing the gastrointestinal tract

_____ 4. Immediately under the skin (SubQ, SC, SQ)

_____ 5. Inside the cheek

_____ 6. Into a joint (IA)

_____ 7. Into a vein (IV)

_____ 8. Into an artery (IA)

_____ 9. Into the ear

_____ 10. Into the eye

_____ 11. Into the eye

_____ 12. Into the heart muscle (IC)

_____ 13. Into the nose

_____ 14. Into the space around the spinal cord

_____ 15. Into the top layers of the skin (ID)

_____ 16. Into the urinary bladder

_____ 17. Into the ventricles, or cavities, of the brain

_____ 18. Through the anus

_____ 19. Through the mouth (PO)

_____ 20. Through the skin

_____ 21. Through the skin

_____ 22. Under the gums

_____ 23. Under the tongue (SL)

True or False

_____ 1. For a systemic effect to take place, absorption of the medication must occur.

_____ 2. Liquid medications are always solutions.

_____ 3. All liquid medications may be made palatable by adding flavors and sweetening agents.

_____ 4. Aqueous solutions can be injected into the bloodstream.

_____ 5. Solid medication dosage forms are usually faster-acting than liquid medication dosage forms.

_____ 6. Medications may be absorbed into the bloodstream as very small particles suspended in an aqueous vehicle.

_____ 7. Like gargles, mouthwashes should be swallowed.

_____ 8. Simple syrup contains sucrose, flavoring, and water.

_____ 9. The only uses for enemas are to relieve severe constipation or to clean the large bowel before surgery.

_____ 10. Elixirs and spirits are examples of hydroalcoholic solutions.

_____ 11. Elixirs should be avoided by alcoholics.

_____ 12. Tablets that are enteric coated should not be crushed, chewed, or cut.

_____ 13. Suppositories may treat local conditions in the immediate area of administration or may exert systemic effects elsewhere.

_____ 14. If it seems necessary to crush, chew, or cut an extended-release product, an immediate-release formulation of the same drug should be used instead.

_____ 15. Continuous infusions may be given by IV push.

Fill in the Blank

1. A _____ effect refers to an action of a medication that takes place at the area of contact.

2. A _____ effect is the result of an action of a medication that affects the whole body or takes place at a location distant from the medication's initial point of contact.

3. _____ are alcoholic or hydroalcoholic solutions whose potency is adjusted so that each milliliter of tincture contains the equivalent of 100 mg of crude drug.

4. _____ contain the equivalent of 1,000 mg of crude drug.

5. _____ are mixtures of two liquids that normally do not mix.

6. _____ tablets contain ingredients that bubble and release the active drug when placed in a liquid.

7. When powders are wetted, allowed to dry, and ground into coarse pieces, the resulting medication dosage form is called a _____.

8. _____ are mixtures of fine particles of an undissolved solid spread throughout a gas or, more commonly, a liquid.

9. _____ are thick, viscous, gummy liquids composed of water that contains the sticky, pulpy parts of vegetables.

10. _____ tablets are placed inside the pouch of the cheek and stick to the inside lining of the cheek.

11. The oral route is abbreviated _____.

12. _____ routes of administration are those that bypass the gastrointestinal tract.

Short Answer

1. Discuss the advantages and disadvantages of liquid medications.

2. Explain the different types of emulsions, including the contents, and the advantages and disadvantages of each type of emulsion.

3. Discuss the uses of the ingredients in compressed tablets that have no medicinal activity.

4. Explain the primary ointment bases and discuss their uses.

5. Discuss the advantages and disadvantages of extended-release products.

Alphabet Soup

For each of the abbreviations below, indicate their meaning.

a. CD

b. CR

c. CRT

d. LA

e. SA

f. SR

g. TD

h. TR

i. XL

j. XR

Crossword Puzzle

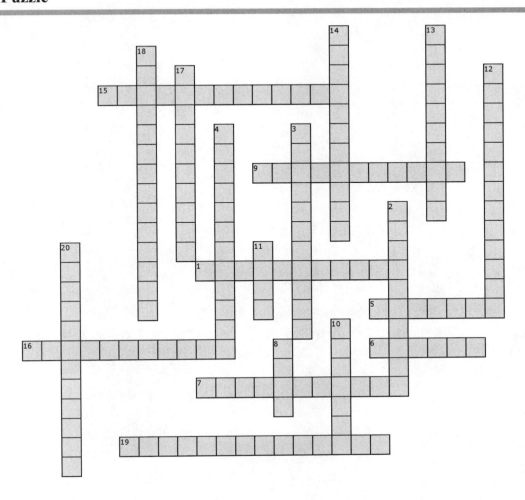

Across:

1. Into the space around the spinal cord
5. By way of the intestine
6. Inside the cheek
7. Under the gums
9. A feeding tube inserted through the abdominal wall into the stomach
15. Into a muscle
16. Into a vein
19. Into a joint

Down:

2. Under the tongue
3. A feeding tube inserted through the nose into the stomach
4. Through the skin
8. Into the ear
10. Applied to skin or mucous membranes
11. Through the mouth
12. Into an artery
13. Into the eye
14. Into the top layers of the skin
17. Bypassing the gastrointestinal tract
18. Into the urinary bladder
20. Immediately under the skin

Chapter 13

Processing Medication Orders and Prescriptions

Learning Outcomes

This chapter reinforces the following learning outcomes discussed in Chapter 13/ Processing Medication Orders and Prescriptions of the *Manual for Pharmacy Technicians, 4th edition.*

- Identify the components of a complete prescription or medication order.
- Prioritize prescriptions and medication orders on the basis of pertinent criteria.
- Describe the necessary steps in processing a prescription or medication order.
- List the information that is typically contained in a patient profile.
- Identify the information that is necessary to make a medication label complete.

Multiple Choice 76

Matching 77

True or False 77

Fill in the Blank 78

Short Answer 78

Alphabet Soup 78

Multiple Choice

1. Medication orders may come to the pharmacy:

   a. Delivered to the pharmacy via hand off or pneumatic tube.
   b. Faxed to the pharmacy.
   c. Scanned to the pharmacy.
   d. All of the above.
   e. None of the above.

2. Medication orders should be prioritized on the basis of a number of factors, including:

   a. The time the medication is needed.
   b. The seriousness of the condition that is being treated.
   c. The urgency of the other medication orders waiting to be processed.
   d. All of the above.
   e. None of the above.

3. Steps involved in processing an order include:

   a. Comparison of the order against the patient's existing medication profile.
   b. Order entry steps.
   c. Selection, preparation, or compounding of medication.
   d. Final check and dispensing of medication.
   e. All of the above.
   f. None of the above.

4. The method to ensure that orders are marked with the correct patient name is to:

   a. Check to see that the order makes sense for the patient by checking the order against the patient profile.
   b. Double checking the patient account number.
   c. Double checking the patient medical record number.
   d. All of the above.
   e. None of the above.

5. Many computer systems offer alerts for:

   a. Drug interactions.
   b. Therapeutic duplications.
   c. Drug allergies.
   d. Over or under the recommended dose.
   e. All of the above.
   f. None of the above.

6. Standardized schedules of drug administration are usually based on:

   a. Physician orders.
   b. Pharmacy hours of operation.
   c. Nursing break times.
   d. All of the above.
   e. None of the above.

7. Odd dosages:

   a. Should be double checked with a pharmacist.
   b. May indicate a prescribing error.
   c. All of the above.
   d. None of the above.

8. When multiple dosage forms of the drug may make sense for an order, considerations might include:

   a. Whether or not a patient can swallow pills.
   b. Whether the patient would prefer to chew tablets.
   c. Whether the patient would prefer to take a liquid medication.
   d. All of the above.
   e. None of the above.

9. Many institutions have developed protocols in which the pharmacist is requested to dose and monitor certain medications. Examples of pharmacist protocols include:

   a. Blood pressure medications.
   b. COPD medications.
   c. Aminoglycoside dosing and monitoring.
   d. All of the above.
   e. None of the above.

10. There are state-by-state variations regarding:

    a. Who can receive a telephone order.
    b. If facsimile transmission is legal for controlled substances.
    c. If e-prescribing is allowed.
    d. All of the above.
    e. None of the above.

Matching

Indicate whether the information below is required in these locations:

A. Inpatient MAR   B.   Outpatient prescription label   C.   Neither

_____ 1. Patient name

_____ 2. Patient account number

_____ 3. Patient birth date

_____ 4. Patient allergies

_____ 5. Brand drug name

_____ 6. Route of administration

_____ 7. Dosage form

_____ 8. Dose/strength

_____ 9. Frequency and duration of administration (if duration is pertinent; may be open-ended)

_____ 10. Indication for use of the medication

_____ 11. Other instructions for the person administering the medication, such as whether it should be given with food or on an empty stomach

_____ 12. Prescriber's name/signature and credentials

_____ 13. Date the order was written

_____ 14. Time the order was written

_____ 15. Sex

_____ 16. Height and weight

_____ 17. Lab values such as serum creatinine

_____ 18. Room and bed number

_____ 19. Quantity to be dispensed

_____ 20. Number of refills to be allowed

_____ 21. Substitution authority or refusal

_____ 22. DEA number for controlled medications

Part 3

True or False

_____ 1. If information is missing from a medication order or an order is unclear, most clarifications can be handled by the pharmacy technician.

_____ 2. An order for phenylephrine, a medication used intravenously to maintain blood pressure in critically ill patients, would usually receive priority over an order for an orally administered vitamin.

_____ 3. Medications ordered for the initial treatment of pain, fever, or nausea and vomiting are generally high priority because of the desire to relieve the patient's discomfort.

_____ 4. A patient's account number never changes, but medical record numbers change every time a patient is admitted to an institution.

_____ 5. It is recommended that prescribers order drug products by brand name instead of generic name.

_____ 6. Default time schedules may differ on some specialized nursing units.

_____ 7. The last step in the order entry process is generally an acceptance (also called verification or validation) function in which the pharmacist verifies that the order is correctly entered for the right patient and is clinically appropriate.

_____ 8. If an inpatient is taking his medications brought in from home, there is no need to enter these medications into the computer system since the patient will not be charged for the medications.

_____ 9. With CPOE, it is not necessary for a pharmacist to review and verify the order before the medication is dispensed because the physician has entered the order.

_____ 10. In all states, when a prescriber signs his or her name over the DAW signature line, the medication must be dispensed as written.

_____ 11. In the outpatient setting, prescriptions are always filled in the order in which they are presented to the pharmacy, and many pharmacies use some type of "take-a-number" system to be entirely fair.

_____ 12. As long as the correct drug is selected regarding medication name and strength, it is not necessary to match the NDC number with the product dispensed, especially when generic products are used.

_____ 13. Unlike inpatient pharmacies, there are no formulary issues in the outpatient setting.

_____ 14. A pharmacist check is legally required in most cases, and must occur before any drug is dispensed to a patient care area.

Fill in the Blank

1. Typically, the term _____ _____ refers to a physician's written, electronic, telephone, or verbal request for a medication in an inpatient setting.

2. The term _____ refers to a medication order on a prescription blank that is transmitted in writing, via oral communication, or by electronic means to be filled in an outpatient or ambulatory care setting.

3. Medication orders may be entered directly into the computer system by the prescriber, which is commonly referred to as computer physician order entry, or _____.

4. The _____ is the part of the patient's medical record in which the caregiver (generally the nurse) documents when medications ordered for a patient are administered.

5. The drug buspirone written as "busPIRone" is an example of a safety precaution utilizing _____ _____ _____.

6. Robotics is an example of automated dispensing products that are located in a _____ location.

7. Robotics or carousel systems use _____ _____ to identify medications accurately during filling.

8. Most prescriptions are now electronically filed with a third-party payer at the time they are entered into the pharmacy information system; this is called electronic claims _____.

9. A label affixed to a drug product that alerts users to special handling or administration concern is called an _____ label.

10. A _____ is a shorthand name for a drug product that facilitates faster computer data entry.

Short Answer

1. Identify the components of a complete prescription or medication order.

2. Discuss the considerations when prioritizing prescriptions and medication orders.

3. Describe the necessary steps in processing a prescription or medication order.

4. List the information that is typically contained in a patient profile.

5. Describe the process of medication management using a decentralized automated dispensing model.

Alphabet Soup

a. CPOE

b. MAR

c. eMAR

d. STAT

e. ASAP

f. QA

g. DAW

h. DNS

i. NDC

j. DEA

Chapter 14

Pharmacy Calculations

Learning Outcomes

This chapter reinforces the following learning outcomes discussed in Chapter 14/ Pharmacy Calculations of the *Manual for Pharmacy Technicians, 4th edition.*

- Explain why it is important to follow a standardized approach when using math in pharmacy.
- Convert between fractions, decimals, and percentages.
- Convert between different systems of measurement.
- Perform and check key pharmacy calculations, including the calculations needed to interpret prescriptions and those involving patient-specific information.

Multiple Choice 80

Matching 81

True or False 82

Fill in the Blank 82

Short Answer 82

Crossword Puzzle 83

Multiple Choice

1. When adding fractions, the three steps in the correct order are:

   a. Reduce to the simplest fractions or mixed numbers, add numerators and denominators, express answer as a fraction and simplify.
   b. Convert to common denominators, add the numerators, reduce to the simplest fractions or mixed numbers.
   c. Convert to common numerators, add denominators, reduce to the simplest fractions.
   d. Add numerators, add denominators, express answer as a fraction and simplify.

2. When multiplying fractions, the steps in the correct order are:

   a. Convert to common denominators, multiply the numerators, express answer as a fraction and simplify.
   b. Multiply the denominators, multiply the numerators, express answer as a fraction and simplify.
   c. Convert to common numerators, multiply the denominators, express answer as a fraction and simplify.
   d. Convert to common denominators, multiply numerators and denominators, express answer as a fraction and simplify.

3. Percentage means:

   a. per each.
   b. per 10.
   c. per 100.
   d. per 1000.

4. The standard units used in health care are:

   a. Meter (distance), liter (mass), gram (volume).
   b. Meter (distance), millimeter (mass), gram (volume).
   c. Centimeter (distance), microgram (volume), milliliter (mass).
   d. Meter (distance), liter (volume), gram (mass).

5. One dram is used to represent:

   a. 5 mL.
   b. 1 teaspoon.
   c. All of the above.
   d. None of the above.

6. Examples of patient-specific calculations that may influence drug dosing include:

   a. Body surface area.
   b. Ideal body weight.
   c. Body mass index.
   d. All of the above.
   e. None of the above.

7. Which of the following statements about BSA values is not true?

   a. BSA values are frequently used to calculate doses of chemotherapeutic agents.
   b. There is one formula that is used to calculate BSA.
   c. Hospital computer systems will usually calculate the BSA value.
   d. It is it is helpful to understand how the calculation is performed.

8. When calculating days' supply for an ophthalmic solution, assume 1 mL =

   a. 10 drops.
   b. 15 drops.
   c. 20 drops.
   d. 25 drops.

9. When mixtures are created by adding a solid to a liquid, the percentage strength is measured in:

   a. Weight in volume (w/v) or grams of drug per 1 mL of mixture.
   b. Volume in weight (v/w) or liters of drug per 100 grams of mixture.
   c. Weight in volume (w/v) or grams of drug per 100 mL of mixture.
   d. Volume in weight (v/w) or milliliters of drug per 10 grams of mixture.

10. The concentrations of very weak solutions are sometimes expressed as ratio strengths. Ratio strengths are usually expressed as 1:something, where the units are:

    a. mg per L.
    b. g per 100 mL.
    c. g per L.
    d. g per mL.

Matching

Match the following terms with the correct definitions.

A. Alligation method

B. Apothecary system

C. Avoirdupois system

D. Body mass index (BMI)

E. Body surface area (BSA)

F. Days supply

G. Denominator

H. Fraction

I. Household system

J. Ideal body weight (IBW)

K. Metric system

L. Numerator

M. Proportion

N. Ratio

O. Ratio strengths

_____ 1. A combination of two ratios with the same units; a statement of equality between two ratios

_____ 2. A French system of mass that includes ounces and pounds

_____ 3. A measure of body fat based on height and weight used to determine if a patient is underweight, of normal weight, overweight, or obese

_____ 4. A part of a whole number used to express quantities less than one or quantities between two whole numbers

_____ 5. A ratio expressed as 1:something, where the units are g per mL. The concentrations of weak solutions such as 1:1000 or 1:10,000 epinephrine are sometimes expressed this way

_____ 6. A representation of the relationship between two items

_____ 7. A system of measurement commonly used in cooking, including the teaspoon, the tablespoon, and the cup

_____ 8. A system of measurement originally developed in Greece for use by physicians and pharmacists but now largely replaced by the metric system

_____ 9. A way to help determine how many parts of each strength should be mixed together to prepare the desired strength

_____ 10. An estimate of how much a patient should weigh based on his or her height and gender; expressed in kg

_____ 11. The time a specific amount of medication will last

_____ 12. The bottom number of a fraction, representing the total number of parts

_____ 13. The most widely used and accepted system of measurement in the world; based on multiples of ten

_____ 14. The top number of a fraction, representing the number of parts present

_____ 15. The total surface area of the body, taking the patient's weight and height into account and expressed in m2

True or False

_____ 1. Numbers to the right of the decimal point represent whole numbers, and numbers to the left of the decimal point represent quantities less than one.

_____ 2. With respect to rounding, pharmacy numbers must be measurable and practical.

_____ 3. Percentages also convert simply to decimals. Just remove the % sign and move the decimal point two places to the left.

_____ 4. The symbol μ has been used as an abbreviation for micro, but this is an unsafe symbol because it can be confused with an "m."

_____ 5. The avoirdupois system is a Spanish system of mass that includes grams and liters.

_____ 6. Ideal body weight (IBW) is an estimate of how much a patient should weigh, based on his or her height and gender and is expressed as pounds.

_____ 7. Body mass index (BMI) is a measure of body fat based on height and weight and is commonly used in medication calculations.

_____ 8. Specific gravity is the ratio of the weight of the compound to the weight of the same amount of water.

_____ 9. Specific gravity is expressed in grams.

_____ 10. In pharmacy calculations, specific gravity and density are used interchangeably.

_____ 11. When calculating concentration percentages of medications, if the product does not contain active ingredient, its concentration is 0%; if the product is pure active ingredient, its concentration is 100%.

_____ 12. Some pharmacy mixtures are created by adding two solids together. When this occurs, the percentage strength is measured in weight in weight (w/w) or grams of drug/10 grams of mixture.

Fill in the Blank

1. The Roman numeral for 10 is _____.

2. The Roman numeral for 50 is _____.

3. The Roman numeral for 100 is _____.

4. The Roman numeral for 5 is _____.

5. The Roman numeral for 1000 is _____.

6. The Roman numeral for ½ is _____.

7. A fraction is written as two whole numbers separated by a division line, for example, ¾. The number on top, or the _____, represents the number of parts present and the number on the bottom, or the_____, represents the total number of parts.

8. A _____ shows the relationship between two items.

9. When the desired concentration of a product is not readily available, but concentrations above and below the desired concentration are available, the _____ method will help to determine how many parts of each strength should be mixed together to prepare the desired strength.

10. The _____ system of measurement was originally developed in Greece for use by physicians and pharmacists and used measurements such as the grain and the dram.

Short Answer

1. Explain the steps in calculating Roman numerals.

2. Explain the steps in adding fractions.

3. Explain the steps in multiplying fractions.

4. Explain the steps in dividing fractions.

5. Discuss BMI, IBW, and BSA.

Crossword Puzzle

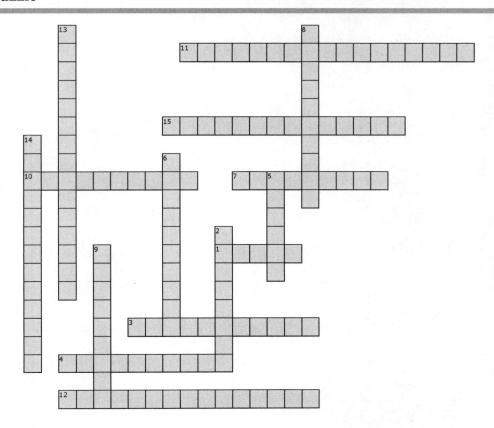

Across:

1. A representation of the relationship between two items. For example, when calculating a dose, a ratio can be used to show the number of milligrams in the dose per one kilogram of patient weight

3. The bottom number of a fraction, representing the total number of parts

4. A combination of two ratios with the same units; a statement of equality between two ratios

7. The top number of a fraction, representing the number of parts present

10. The amount of medication dispensed for a specified time period

11. A French system of mass that includes ounces and pounds; the system of mass most commonly utilized in the United States

12. The total surface area of the body, taking the patient's weight and height into account and expressed in m2

15. A ratio expressed as 1:something, where the units are g per mL. The concentrations of weak solutions such as 1:1000 or 1:10,000 epinephrine are sometimes expressed this way

Down:

2. A part of a whole number used to express quantities less than one or quantities between two whole numbers

5. The most widely used and accepted system of measurement in the world; based on multiples of ten

6. A way to help determine how many parts of each strength should be mixed together to prepare the desired strength

8. A system of measurement, originally developed in Greece for use by physicians and pharmacists but now largely replaced by the metric system, including the grain and the dram, the most common apothecary measures seen today

9. A system of measurement commonly used in cooking, including the teaspoon, the tablespoon, and the cup

13. An estimate of how much a patient should weigh based on his or her height and gender; expressed in kg

14. A measure of body fat based on height and weight, used to determine if a patient is underweight, of normal weight, overweight, or obese

Chapter 15

Nonsterile Compounding and Repackaging

Learning Outcomes

This chapter reinforces the following learning outcomes discussed in Chapter 15/Nonsterile Compounding and Repackaging of the *Manual for Pharmacy Technicians, 4th edition.*

- Define compounding.
- Describe the steps involved in the compounding process.
- Describe the equipment commonly used when compounding preparations.
- Identify the types of preparations commonly compounded.
- Explain the concept of and reasons for repackaging medications.
- Explain the importance of record keeping for compounding and repackaging.

Multiple Choice 86

Matching 87

True or False 88

Fill in the Blank 89

Short Answer 89

Word Search 90

Multiple Choice

1. Compounding is often associated with several specialty practice areas, including:

   a. Veterinary medicine.
   b. Dermatology.
   c. Hormone replacement therapy.
   d. All of the above.
   e. None of the above.

2. The compounding environment should:

   a. Have adequate space for the orderly placement and storage of equipment and support materials.
   b. Have controlled temperature and lighting.
   c. Be kept clean for sanitary reasons and to prevent cross contamination.
   d. All of the above.
   e. None of the above.

3. Primary packaging of the finished medication is of utmost importance. The choice of the proper container is guided by the physical and chemical characteristics of the finished medication. Examples of container choices to maximize stability should take into consideration:

   a. Whether the medication is light sensitive.
   b. If the medication binds to the container.
   c. All of the above.
   d. None of the above.

4. Things to consider for determining beyond-use dates include whether:

   a. The medication is aqueous (water-based) or non-aqueous.
   b. A technician or a pharmacist compounded the mixture.
   c. The medication is comprised of legend medications.
   d. All of the above.
   e. None of the above.

5. Each step of the compounding process should be documented in order to:

   a. Allow another individual to reproduce the same formulation at a later date.
   b. Calculate charges.
   c. Look for ways to improve efficiency.
   d. All of the above.
   e. None of the above.

6. The compounding record is the log of an actual compounded preparation or batch being prepared and includes:

   a. Manufacturer and lot numbers of chemicals used, the date of preparation, and an internal identification number.
   b. A beyond-use date.
   c. The names of the individuals who prepared and verified the preparation.
   d. All of the above.
   e. None of the above.

7. When using a graduate, it is recommended:

   a. To use glass graduates rather than plastic graduates.
   b. To use conicals rather than cylinders.
   c. To use the smallest graduate that will hold the volume to be measured.
   d. All of the above.
   e. None of the above.

8. Mortars and pestles are used to crush, grind, and blend various medicinal ingredients. Which of the following statements regarding mortars and pestles is true?

   a. The mortar is the "bowl," and the pestle is the "stirrer."
   b. The pestle is the "bowl," and the mortar is the "stirrer."
   c. Mortar and pestle refer to the set of the "bowl" and the "stirrer," and each piece is not individually named.

9. With regard to levigation agents,

   a. Mineral oil is always used because of its versatility.
   b. Glycerin is always used because it has no effect on the final product.
   c. Compatibility in the final preparation is considered in the selection.
   d. Any moist substance may be used, since only a tiny amount is used.

10. The main task of an ointment mill is to:

    a. Blend the various ingredients.
    b. Fill ointment tubes efficiently.
    c. Keep the compounding area organized.
    d. Reduce particle size in preparations.

Matching

A. Active ingredient

B. Batch record

C. Batch repackaging

D. Beyond-use labeling

E. Blister packages

F. Compounding

G. Compounding environment

H. Extemporaneous repackaging

I. Geometric dilution

J. Graduates

K. Inactive ingredient

L. Levigation

M. Manufacturing

N. Nonsterile compounding

O. Peristaltic pumps

P. Prescription compounding

Q. Stability

R. Sterile compounding

S. Trituration

T. Unit-dose package

U. Volumetric pumps

_____ 1. A compounding method of incorporating a solid into an ointment. A small amount of a levigating agent is added to the powder to form a paste, which is then incorporated into the ointment.

_____ 2. A date that is given to a medication noting when it should no longer be used; also referred to as the expiration date.

_____ 3. A medication individualized for a specific patient that requires the mixing of ingredients in a pharmacy and is based on a prescription or drug order.

_____ 4. A non-reusable container designed to hold a quantity of drug to be administered as a single dose.

_____ 5. An ingredient that is necessary to prepare the formulation, but is not intended to cause a pharmacologic response.

_____ 6. Compounding equipment used to measure the volume of liquid ingredients; generally glass or plastic cylinders and conicals.

_____ 7. Compounding technique used to ensure the uniform mixing when there is a wide discrepancy in amounts of individual ingredients.

_____ 8. Compounds prepared in a pharmacy that do not require strict aseptic technique and include preparations such as oral and topical medications.

_____ 9. Compounds prepared in a pharmacy using strict aseptic technique, including preparations such as injections, ophthalmic solutions, and irrigation solutions.

_____ 10. Defined in USP-NF as the extent to which a preparation retains, within specified limits and throughout its period of storage and use, the same properties and characteristics that it possessed at the time of compounding.

_____ 11. Includes the facilities (i.e., compounding area) and equipment in the pharmacy.

_____ 12. Ingredient in the compounded preparation that is responsible for the therapeutic or pharmaceutical action of the medication.

_____ 13. Often called "bubble packs." Composed of a plastic bubble that forms a cavity for the medication. The package is then sealed with a backing material that also acts as a label.

_____ 14. Pumps that allow the user to preset a volume to be dispensed into a container on the basis of the draw back setting.

_____ 15. Pumps with a series of roller wheels that press against tubing to force a volume of liquid down the length of the tubing.

_____ 16. Repackaging quantities of medications that will be used within a short period of time.

_____ 17. The act of mixing powders or crushing tablets using a mortar and pestle until a state of fine, evenly sized particles is achieved.

_____ 18. The compounding record for a batch, usually filed by lot number.

_____ 19. The periodic repackaging of large quantities of medications in unit-dose or single-unit packages.

_____ 20. Typically occurs in licensed manufacturing facilities and includes the production, conversion, and/or processing of a drug, generally in bulk quantities and without a prescription or medication order.

_____ 21. Usually takes place in a pharmacy and includes the preparation, mixing, packaging, and labeling of a small quantity of a drug based on a practitioner's prescription or medication order for a specific patient.

True or False

_____ 1. When pharmacies compound both sterile and nonsterile preparations, the compounding area for sterile preparations is also used for compounding nonsterile preparations.

_____ 2. If a patient needs a drug that has been withdrawn from the market by the FDA, the patient should ask a compounding pharmacy to order the ingredients and compound the medication.

_____ 3. Preparations should contain at least 90%, but not more than 110%, of the labeled active ingredient, unless more restrictive guidelines apply.

_____ 4. To be as efficient as possible, several similar preparations may be compounded at one time in the compounding area if the compounding personnel are experienced.

_____ 5. Patient counseling is not required for compounded medications.

_____ 6. Because they do not cause pharmacologic activity, inactive ingredients are not a necessary part of the product, and the specific chemicals used as excipients do not need to be named in the formula.

_____ 7. Once a class A torsion balance is calibrated, it does not need to be recalibrated as long as it remains on a stable and solid surface.

_____ 8. The bottom of the meniscus should be read at counter level.

_____ 9. Wedgewood mortars are preferable when mixing liquids or preparing solutions, suspensions, or lotions, adding flavoring oils and coloring.

_____ 10. An ointment slab or ointment paper may be used for preparing and mixing creams and ointments.

_____ 11. Numerous capsule sizes and colors are available for human and veterinary use. Sizes of capsules for humans range from No. 000 to No. 5. No. 000 is the smallest, and No. 5 is the largest.

_____ 12. Extemporaneous repackaging is also known as "just-in-time" packaging.

_____ 13. End-product testing is performed for all repackaging processes.

_____ 14. Peristaltic pumps need less recalibrating than volumetric pumps and are more accurate and reliable for delivering fluid volumes of less than 10 mL.

Fill in the Blank

1. The United States Pharmacopeia and The National Formulary (USP-NF) offers guidelines and an enforceable set of standards describing procedures and requirements for compounding in Chapter _____ (Pharmaceutical Compounding–Nonsterile Preparations).

2. _____ is defined in USP-NF as "the extent to which a preparation retains, within specified limits, and throughout its period of storage and use, the same properties and characteristics that it possessed at the time of compounding."

3. The _____ date is the date after which a preparation is not to be used and is calculated from the date it was compounded.

4. Each step of the compounding process should be documented. USP Chapter 795 requires pharmacies to maintain a formulation record, also known as the _____ _____, and a compounding record for each compounded preparation.

5. The _____ is the natural curvature of the surface of the liquid, and it is lower in the middle than at the edges.

6. Mixing powders or crushing tablets by moving the pestle in a circular motion in the mortar until a state of fine, evenly sized particles is achieved is termed _____.

7. Before incorporating a powder into the ointment, a paste is first formed by adding a small amount (sufficient to form a paste) of an appropriate agent such as mineral oil. Particle size is then reduced by rubbing the paste on the ointment slab/paper using a spatula. This method of incorporating a solid into the ointment is termed _____.

8. _____ _____ is a technique that is used to ensure the uniform mixing of various amounts of different ingredients and is used when there is a wide discrepancy in amounts of individual ingredients.

9. The _____ _____ _____ is a unique three-segment number that is used to identify a specific drug product.

10. _____ repackaging is repackaging quantities of medications that will be used within a short period of time.

11. _____ repackaging is the periodic repackaging of large quantities of medications in unit-dose or single-unit packages.

12. _____ are the steps in the repackaging process that are crucial to ensuring a high-quality package.

Short Answer

1. Discuss the steps in the nonsterile compounding process.

2. Discuss the considerations when choosing a mortar and pestle for compounding a mixture.

3. Discuss compounding records. Who mandates compounding records and what information must be documented?

4. Discuss beyond-use dating and labeling requirements for repackaged medications.

Part 3

Word Search

```
G S F O R M U L A T I O N R E C O R D M C I T R U
E T A G I V E L L L G N I I G A K C A P E R I I D
E L O C I I I I Q M S U O E N A R O P M E T X E C
S B I I R M C E M P O E N D U N G G L D O R T X L
S R A R T E S I N G G Y T E L I B A T S F A S T N
N A O T E U C A M C N E S T A B I L I T Y I T A T
I S I C N T E O V O L U M E T R I C P U M P S C S
O S U M I E S G N I G A K C A P E R L I G N U R S
P Y N O A L D R O C E R N I O T A L U M R O F N G
K E E O O N I P P E R I S T A L T I C P U M P S A
C G R X I I U R I V O L U M E T R I C P U U R T A
E N S I T T N F R C O M P O U N D I N G G R U R I
H I E L S E A E A I N S T E R A L E N C E R I I R
C D L M E T M L N C G R L E V I G A T I O F T T M
D N A A A U A P O D T A U E I E N T I I E G R U R
P U O C D N Q L O S P U T T V T E I R A P E I R F
U O I I O C U I T R N R R I C I I I E O N O T A G
N P O R T M P F N I A E O I O A G R S U C M U T S
O M D I U A P T A H C N I D N N F A E I P E R I E
I O S N C Q G O U C C P E T U G S U T S B T A O R
T C T T P M L I U E T E U U I C C O N R D R T N E
U E S S A N I U V N M U T P S G T N L A E I I E C
L L G E I B V A A E D L I C S N I P I U M C O A P
I I S T T L I D R E L L S N I I T R S U T D I I N
C R O A T U G L O P P O T U G T I R R C E I T P S
I E I U U X A I P R A O N A K S P T E I I L O U U
R T U D K E T D I R I I I U U E T E M D I U I N I
T S D A D E O P A P I C O D R T I G S M S T R H S
E N L R E N I T T R A I P A F K S T R A V I G P E
M O P G M A N D R C G R K R C R A N E S T O N E L
E N I T E O T N O E G N C G C I I R T P M N E T L
O O T N E I D E R G N I E V I T C A N I D E N G G
G E N D P R O D T A N S H I T R I T U R A T O E N
N D I N A T P I L R G E C I I D A O E A B C I C T
```

ASEPTICTECHNIQUE

CHECKPOINTS

COMPOUNDING

ENDPRODUCT

EXTEMPORANEOUS

FORMULATIONRECORD

GEOMETRICDILUTION

GRADUATES

INACTIVEINGREDIENT

IRRIGATIONSOLUTIONS

LEVIGATION

MANUFACTURING

NONSTERILECOMPOUNDING

PERISTALTICPUMPS

REPACKAGING

STABILITY

STERILE

TESTING

TRITURATION

VOLUMETRICPUMPS

Chapter 16

Aseptic Technique, Sterile Compounding, and IV Admixture Programs

Learning Outcomes

This chapter reinforces the following learning outcomes discussed in Chapter 16/
Aseptic Technique, Sterile Compounding, and IV Admixture Programs of the
Manual for Pharmacy Technicians, 4th edition.

- Describe the basics of intravenous drug therapy.
- Describe the key elements of working in laminar airflow workbenches.
- List the common types of contamination that may occur when working in a
  laminar flow hood and describe how to minimize the risks of these types of
  contamination.
- Perform basic manipulations needed to prepare a sterile product by using asep-
  tic technique.
- Describe the risks of handling cytotoxic and hazardous drugs.
- List the steps in drug preparation and handling that are unique to cytotoxic and
  hazardous drugs.
- List the typical ingredients of a total parenteral nutrition solution.
- Describe the manual and automated means of preparing total parenteral nutri-
  tion solutions.
- Describe the benefits of having a formal intravenous admixture program.
- Describe how USP 797 has impacted the preparation of sterile products.

Multiple Choice 92

Matching 93

True or False 93

Fill in the Blank 94

Short Answer 94

Crossword Puzzle 95

Multiple Choice

1. IV administration of medications is beneficial because:

    a. There is a rapid onset of action.
    b. Patients who are unconscious can be medicated.
    c. Patients who are nauseated can be medicated.
    d. All of the above.
    e. None of the above.

2. Infection from IV administration of medications may be due to contamination during:

    a. Preparation.
    b. Administration.
    c. Improper storage.
    d. All of the above.
    e. None of the above.

3. Particulate matter in IVs may include:

    a. Microscopic glass fragments, hair, lint, or cotton fibers.
    b. Undissolved drug particles.
    c. Fragments of rubber stoppers.
    d. All of the above.
    e. None of the above.

4. Phlebitis, or irritation of the vein, is caused by:

    a. The IV catheter or the location of the IV site.
    b. The drug being administered (due to its chemical properties or its concentration) or too fast a rate of administration.
    c. The presence of particulate matter.
    d. All of the above.
    e. None of the above.

5. The concentration of heparin used in heparin locks is usually:

    a. 1 unit/mL or 10 units/mL.
    b. 10 units/mL or 100 units/mL.
    c. 100 units/mL or 1000 units/mL.
    d. 1000 units/mL or 10,000 units/mL.

6. The final filter constitutes the entire back portion of the hood's work area, and this filter is called a:

    a. High efficiency particulate air or HEPA filter.
    b. Horizontal exhaust pressure area or HEPA filter.
    c. Hazardous elimination processing activator or HEPA filter.
    d. Laminar airflow filter (LAFF).

7. It is advisable to work with objects at least _____ from the sides and front edge of the hood without blocking air vents, so that unobstructed airflow is maintained between the HEPA filter and sterile objects.

    a. 4 inches
    b. 6 inches
    c. 8 inches
    d. 10 inches

8. When a LAFW has been turned off and is turned back on, it should be allowed to run for _____ minutes before it is used in order to blow the non-sterile air out of the LAFW work area.

    a. 5-10
    b. 10-15
    c. 15-30
    d. 30-60

9. Before use, all interior working surfaces of the laminar flow workbench should be cleaned with _____ isopropyl alcohol or other appropriate disinfecting agent and a clean, lint-free cloth.

    a. 50%
    b. 70%
    c. 90%
    d. 99%

10. The side walls of the hood should be cleaned in a(n):

    a. Side-to-side direction, starting at the HEPA and working toward the outer edge of the hood.
    b. Side-to-side direction, starting at the outer edge and working toward the HEPA filter in the hood.
    c. Up-and-down direction, starting at outer edge and working toward the HEPA filter in the hood.
    d. Up-and-down direction, starting at the HEPA and working toward the outer edge of the hood.

Matching

Match the ingredients of a TPN to the correct general class; some general classes will be used more than once.

A. Carbohydrate

B. Electrolyte

C. Lipid

D. Protein

E. Vitamin

_____ 1. Dextrose

_____ 2. Amino acids

_____ 3. Sodium chloride

_____ 4. Potassium chloride

_____ 5. Potassium phosphate

_____ 6. Calcium gluconate

_____ 7. Magnesium sulfate

_____ 8. MVI

_____ 9. 10% fat emulsion

_____ 10. Vitamin K

True or False

_____ 1. IVs may be administered to patients at home by their families rather than by nurses.

_____ 2. When drugs are injected directly into the body, the body's barriers to infection are bypassed.

_____ 3. Drug incompatibilities may involve other drugs, containers, or solutions.

_____ 4. Extravasation is a very minor problem, seldom causing any complications.

_____ 5. When an IV solution is sterilized, pyrogens are removed.

_____ 6. When drugs are added to the IV solution to prepare the final sterile product, the drug is referred to as the admixture and the final product is referred to as the additive.

_____ 7. All laminar flow workbenches should be cleaned with alcohol.

_____ 8. Nothing should be permitted to come in contact with the HEPA filter.

_____ 9. Only those objects essential to product preparation should be placed in the LAFW such as pens and labels.

_____ 10. Jewelry may be worn on the hands or wrists when working in the LAFW as long as appropriate clean room attire covers all exposures.

_____ 11. Every entry into a sterile product area should include scrubbing your hands, nails, wrists, and forearms to elbows thoroughly for at least 30 seconds with a brush, warm water, and appropriate bactericidal soap before performing aseptic manipulations.

_____ 12. Due to their toxicity, solutions with preservatives should not be used for epidural or intrathecal dosage forms and should only be used with caution in pediatric or neonatal preparations.

_____ 13. To withdraw the solution from an ampule, a needle with a 5-micron filter in the hub should be used for withdrawing contents and expelling contents.

_____ 14. All hazardous drugs should be identified by distinctive labels, indicating that the product requires special handling.

_____ 15. Precipitation may occur if the wrong sequence or concentrations of electrolytes are added to an IV bag.

Fill in the Blank

1. A type of catheter that offers some of the benefits of both central and peripheral catheters and is threaded through the venous system and its tip ends near the heart is called a _____ catheter.

2. It is called _____ when the IV catheter punctures and exits the vein under the skin, causing drugs to infuse or infiltrate into the tissue.

3. _____ are the by-products or remnants of bacteria, and they can cause reactions (e.g., fever, chills) if injected in large enough amounts.

4. _____ is irritation of the vein, and it may be caused by the IV catheter, the drug itself due to its chemical properties or its concentration, the location of the IV site, the rate of administration, or the presence of particulate matter.

5. Large volume parenterals are defined as IV solutions greater than _____ mL in volume.

6. Another term for a small volume parenteral IV is _____.

7. The system that uses a specially designed bag and vial where the vial is screwed into a special receptacle on the top of the bag and reconstitution occurs by manipulations done on the outside of the bag and the stopper remains in the bag is called the _____ system.

8. The term _____ is used to refer to pumps designed to alert the user to an infusion setting that does not match a facility's drug administration guidelines, where the medication's infusion parameters such as dose, dosing unit (mcg/kg/min, units/hr, etc.), rate, or concentration can be safely chosen with notification for doses that fall outside the recommended range.

9. A device for medication infusion that is similar in concept to a water balloon inside a plastic bottle where the balloon is filled with drug solution, and the pressure of the container forces it through the tubing, eliminating the need for a separate pump is called a(n) _____ _____ _____.

10. _____ technique is a means of manipulating sterile products without compromising their sterility.

11. Sterile products should be prepared in ISO Class _____ environments, which contain no more than 100 particles per cubic foot that are 0.5 micron or larger in size.

12. In _____ LAFWs, HEPA-filtered air emerges from the top and passes downward through the work area.

13. _____ are single-dose containers composed entirely of glass and, once broken (i.e., opened), become open-system containers.

14. You should refer to USP Chapter_____, "Pharmaceutical Compounding—Sterile Preparations," for a full description of recommendations and regulations regarding IV admixture programs.

Short Answer

1. Discuss the risks involved with IV therapy.

2. Name some simple and inexpensive practices that will reduce the particulate counts in IV rooms.

3. Explain the differences in the types of LAFWs and when each type of LAFW should be used.

4. In some institutions, it is the responsibility of the pharmacy to prime the line with the chemotherapeutic agent. Explain the process.

5. What is a spill kit?

Crossword Puzzle

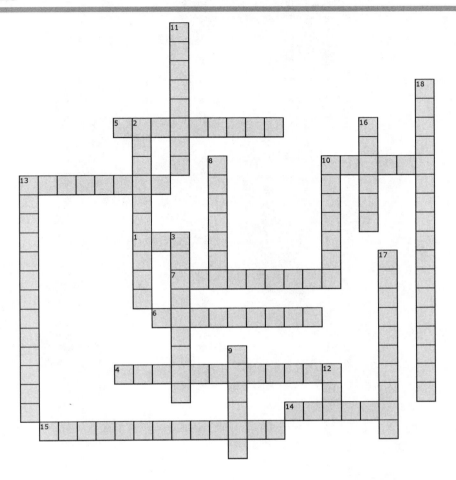

Across:

1. IV solutions greater than 100 mL in volume
4. Needed to meet daily metabolic needs
5. Irritation of the vein
6. Cell killer
7. Causes mutation by damaging DNA
10. Single use glass containers that must be broken for access to medication
13. Administration of drugs involves placing a special catheter into the space of the spine
14. Fats usually administered as fat emulsions
15. Required for proper enzymatic reactions and for use of energy sources in the body

Down:

2. A filter that removes 99.97% of all air particles 0.3 micrometers or larger used in LAFWs
3. Small volume parenteral
8. Required for tissue synthesis and repair
9. Introducing particulate matter in the form of a plastic or rubber "core" or plug into a sterile fluid through the process of penetrating the outer seal of a vial or bag with a needle
10. The technique and procedures designed to prevent contamination of drugs, packaging, equipment, or supplies by microorganisms during preparation
11. The by-products or remnants of bacteria
12. Also called an IV piggyback (IVPB)
13. Results when IV catheter punctures and exits the vein under the skin
16. A quick method to administer some medications
17. A type of system that reduces the risks of needle sticks
18. Procedures that ensure that the processes used in sterile product preparation consistently result in sterile products of acceptable quality

Chapter 17

Medication Errors

Learning Outcomes

This chapter reinforces the following learning outcomes discussed in Chapter 17/
Medication Errors of the *Manual for Pharmacy Technicians, 4th edition.*

- List eleven different types of medication errors.
- Identify causes or factors that contribute to medication errors.
- List five "high alert" medications.
- Describe methods of preventing medication errors from occurring.
- List examples of common medication errors.
- Describe the possible consequences of actual medication errors.
- Explain the steps to be taken when an error has been identified.
- Explain the role of quality assurance monitoring of medication errors.

Multiple Choice 98

Matching 99

True or False 99

Fill in the Blank 100

Short Answer 100

Word Search 101

Multiple Choice

1. Medication error rate comparisons are challenging because of:

   a. The different monitoring, measuring, and reporting techniques used.
   b. Physicians' assistants workload.
   c. Differences in hospitals' census.
   d. All of the above.
   e. None of the above.

2. The Harvard medical practice study that analyzed the incidence of adverse events in hospitalized patients found that ____ of the adverse events that occurred in hospitalized patients were related to drug complications.

   a. None
   b. 9%
   c. 19%
   d. 59%

3. An evaluation of causes of prescribing errors in hospitals found that the majority of potentially serious prescribing errors were made because of:

   a. Lack of knowledge about new drugs and procedures.
   b. Lack of up-to-date references at site of prescribing.
   c. Performance lapses or failure to follow established procedures.
   d. Lack of information about patients such as drug allergies.

4. Medication errors occur:

   a. Only in the pharmacy.
   b. During the prescribing process.
   c. When a nurse transcribes a medication order.
   d. At any point during the medication use process.

5. The list of specific categories of medication errors:

   a. Makes it simple to classify errors.
   b. Defines each possibility clearly so that every error can fall into one of the categories.
   c. Helps to classify errors, but some errors may fit in several of the categories.
   d. Just confuses the process and is not helpful.

6. An unauthorized drug error might occur if:

   a. A medication for one patient was given mistakenly to another patient.
   b. A nurse gave a medication without a prescriber order.

   c. Patients "share" prescriptions at home.
   d. Administration of a medication occurs outside established guidelines.
   e. All of the above.
   f. None of the above.

7. Wrong drug preparation errors include all of the following except:

   a. Reconstituting an azithromycin oral suspension with an incorrect volume of water.
   b. Using bacteriostatic saline instead of sterile water to reconstitute a lyophilized powder for injection.
   c. Not activating an ADD-Vantage® IV admixture bag.
   d. Forgetting to administer the ADD-Vantage® IV admixture bag.

8. When patients read about or experience an adverse drug event, they may:

   a. Lose faith in the medical community.
   b. Choose to switch pharmacies or physicians.
   c. Hesitate to seek medical help for fear of not receiving quality care.
   d. Seek nonconventional treatments from outside the medical community.
   e. All of the above.
   f. None of the above.

9. When a prescription is filled with a wrong strength of a medication because of illegible handwriting, it should be classified as:

   a. Unauthorized drug error.
   b. Improper dose error.
   c. Wrong drug preparation error.
   d. Prescribing error.

10. The Harvard medical practice study that analyzed the incidence of adverse events in hospitalized patients found that _____% of the adverse events that occurred in hospitalized patients were related to drug complications.

   a. 1
   b. 10
   c. 19
   d. 38

Matching

Match the errors with the correct category of error.

A. Prescribing error

B. Omission error

C. Wrong time error

D. Unauthorized drug error

E. Improper dose error

F. Wrong dosage form error

G. Wrong drug preparation error

H. Wrong administration technique error

I. Deteriorated drug error

J. Monitoring error

K. Compliance error

L. No error

_____ 1. Mrs. Jones took her antibiotic for 6 days until she felt better, although she was supposed to take the medication for 10 days.

_____ 2. George was having stomach problems so his neighbor shared his PPI medication because it worked so well for him.

_____ 3. At St. Francis Hospital, all medications must be given within 1 hour of the assigned administration time. Nurse Cratchet gave Bob his 0900 medication at 0800.

_____ 4. Fred was supposed to get 13 units of insulin for a blood glucose reading of 160-170. His BG was 169. He received 12 units of insulin.

_____ 5. Greta was mixing up a bottle of Cleocin Pediatric. She was supposed to add 75 mL of water to make a total of 100 mL of solution. She only added 60 mL of water, so she changed the total quantity to 80 mL and changed the directions to make sure the patient got the correct dose.

_____ 6. Justine forgot to take her vitamin D on Tuesday.

_____ 7. Nurse Annie was supposed to give Frank 100 mg of atenolol each day as long as his blood pressure was greater than 160/100. His blood pressure has been over 160/100 every day for 3 weeks, so she skipped taking the blood pressure reading today and gave him his medication anyway.

_____ 8. The physician prescribed ciprofloxacin for a 7-year-old child. The pharmacist called the physician and reminded him that this class of drugs should be avoided in children.

_____ 9. The physician's directions were for Boric Acid Capsules 500 mg q day. The nurse gave the patient this dose by mouth. The intended route was vaginal.

_____ 10. The expiration date on the bottle of naproxen 500 mg was 7-10. The patient received a prescription of naproxen 500 g #20 1 tab bid on 7-3-10.

True or False

_____ 1. Some of the errors as defined in the ASHP guidelines apply primarily to patients in health care facilities and do not apply to other settings such as home health care, clinic, and physician office settings or outpatient pharmacy practice settings.

_____ 2. There have been numerous and thorough studies of medication errors in hospitals.

_____ 3. Errors occurring earlier in the medication use process (in the prescribing phase) are less likely to be detected and corrected than those occurring later in the process (in administration).

_____ 4. A good general rule to follow is to question any dose that requires less than ½ or more than 2 of the dosage unit (tablet, capsule, teaspoonful).

_____ 5. The recipient of a verbal or telephone order should immediately repeat the order to the prescriber and then immediately write down the order to ensure clarity.

_____ 6. The pharmacist should clarify ambiguous doses before the technician processes the order.

_____ 7. Read the label at least three times to help prevent medication errors: when you remove it from the shelf, as it is being prepared, and as the finished product is set aside for the pharmacist to check.

_____ 8. The abbreviation "qid" is considered unsafe by the Joint Commission.

_____ 9. The correct way to write Coumadin ½ mg using decimals is "Coumadin .5 mg."

_____ 10. The correct way to abbreviate microgram is µg.

Fill in the Blank

1. The term medication _____ is used to describe adverse drug reactions (unintended responses to drugs used at normal doses), adverse drug events (an injury from a medicine or lack of an intended medicine), and medication errors (errors related to the medication use process that may or may not result in adverse drug outcomes).

2. A(n) _____ error occurs at the time a prescriber orders a drug for a specific patient. Errors can include the selection of an incorrect drug, dose, dosage form, route of administration, length of therapy, or number of doses.

3. Failure to administer an ordered dose to a patient in a hospital, long-term care facility, or other facility before the next scheduled dose is considered a(n) _____ error.

4. An institution may determine that administering medications within a specified time of the scheduled time is acceptable, so that medications administered outside this window would be considered _____ _____ errors.

5. A(n) _____ _____ error might occur if a medication for one patient was given mistakenly to another patient or if a nurse gave a medication without a prescriber order.

6. _____ _____ errors occur when a patient is given a dose that is greater or less than the prescribed dose.

7. Doses administered or dispensed in a different form than ordered by the prescriber are classified as _____ _____ _____ errors.

8. Drugs that require reconstitution (adding liquid to dissolve a powdered drug), dilution, or special actions prior to dispensing or administration are subject to _____ _____ _____ errors.

9. Doses that are given to a patient using an inappropriate procedure or incorrect technique are categorized as _____ _____ _____ errors.

10. Medications that are dispensed or administered beyond their expiration date are considered to be _____ _____ errors.

11. _____ errors result from inadequate drug therapy review.

12. Medication errors are committed by patients when they fail to follow or adhere to a prescribed drug regimen; this is referred to as a _____ error.

Short Answer

1. Discuss how workplace issues may affect medication errors.

2. Explain the purpose and procedures for FMEA.

3. What is the purpose of root cause analysis, and when and how would you proceed with one?

4. Calculation errors can lead to serious events. Discuss the errors that are common with calculations and what technicians can do to help reduce the possibility of calculation errors.

Word Search

```
I  H  S  E  T  I  M  P  R  O  P  E  R  D  O  S  E  Z  S  E  I  U  P  R  S
H  S  R  N  U  N  A  U  T  H  O  R  I  Z  E  D  O  N  N  R  S  E  I  D  E
U  R  O  N  S  O  N  G  N  I  R  O  T  I  N  O  M  R  O  E  R  P  R  D  C
U  I  V  I  T  C  E  P  S  O  R  T  E  R  X  N  N  T  I  U  S  E  U  E  N
P  T  R  A  I  L  I  N  G  Z  E  R  O  C  D  U  I  I  T  I  I  D  T  A  I
D  O  S  A  G  E  F  O  R  M  S  I  A  N  F  N  A  N  A  G  I  O  N  C  E
T  I  C  E  I  N  S  U  L  I  A  I  D  N  O  E  E  I  C  N  N  M  E  R  U
O  P  P  R  E  S  C  I  B  I  N  G  S  M  I  V  E  N  I  I  I  I  V  D  I
T  A  P  O  T  H  E  C  A  R  Y  I  M  Y  D  U  I  S  D  R  R  R  D  G  U
D  E  Z  Z  I  R  O  H  T  U  A  N  U  A  L  N  E  U  E  O  A  U  A  M  E
I  I  R  H  I  G  H  A  L  E  R  T  S  M  N  A  R  I  M  O  P  L  S  I  N
E  O  P  M  S  I  G  E  Z  G  N  I  D  A  E  L  N  S  D  T  I  A  I  I  N
D  N  L  I  E  C  O  T  E  L  M  E  T  M  L  M  S  A  E  I  H  I  M  S  O
O  I  E  P  C  U  N  O  I  T  A  C  I  D  E  M  R  E  R  N  E  F  I  T  A
M  T  A  R  O  P  E  S  R  O  O  T  C  A  U  S  E  N  I  O  R  I  Z  N  L
E  A  D  O  M  M  I  E  L  A  H  G  I  H  E  A  O  A  P  M  E  N  D  A  E
R  C  I  P  P  D  I  R  E  R  R  O  R  V  E  C  A  L  X  I  N  I  E  L  E
U  I  N  E  L  C  T  S  O  S  I  U  I  B  I  R  C  S  E  R  P  O  T  U  E
L  D  G  R  I  I  A  L  S  N  N  T  A  H  I  G  H  A  L  I  R  T  E  G  I
I  E  Z  D  A  M  A  D  I  I  C  I  A  P  O  H  E  C  A  R  Y  A  R  A  O
A  M  E  O  E  A  C  L  M  E  O  R  O  O  T  C  A  U  M  R  I  C  I  O  Z
F  D  R  S  S  L  U  I  P  I  R  N  I  T  O  A  I  I  S  O  E  I  O  C  O
E  E  O  E  A  S  C  S  G  S  N  O  I  T  A  L  U  C  L  A  C  D  R  I  S
C  R  A  T  N  Q  O  F  M  N  H  I  D  I  E  L  I  U  S  Z  C  E  A  T  Q
M  I  R  I  S  R  I  I  E  I  I  E  S  M  E  R  U  L  I  A  F  M  T  N  T
G  P  R  E  T  F  S  S  P  D  M  B  P  T  N  D  R  C  Z  U  E  D  E  A  I
E  X  E  E  R  M  S  L  I  R  F  E  I  A  R  O  D  U  L  U  S  E  D  S  N
N  E  R  E  A  E  I  A  A  T  D  O  L  R  L  A  E  L  R  A  M  R  D  H  R
E  I  T  I  A  A  M  M  E  U  Q  I  N  H  C  E  T  S  R  G  C  I  R  A  T
L  A  R  R  O  I  O  I  E  R  R  O  D  N  M  S  Z  I  S  P  S  P  U  G  R
I  I  E  A  E  O  C  C  M  E  D  I  C  A  T  O  E  N  O  I  E  X  G  I  D
I  R  T  F  P  Z  S  E  U  S  E  O  C  T  O  E  R  R  B  N  M  E  H  C  C
M  N  R  N  O  E  A  D  C  O  M  P  L  I  A  N  C  E  P  H  C  O  D  O  O
E  N  Y  L  S  H  H  G  I  V  N  M  I  I  R  E  T  I  E  T  H  H  R  R  F
```

ADMINISTRATION	IMPROPERDOSE
ANALYSIS	INSULIN
ANTICOAGULANTS	ISMP
APOTHECARY	LEADINGZERO
CALCULATIONS	MEDICATION
COMPLIANCE	MISADVENTURE
DECIMALS	MONITORING
DETERIORATEDDRUG	OMISSION
DOSAGEFORM	PRESCRIBING
ERROR	RCA
EXPIREDMEDICATION	RETROSPECTIVE
FAILUREMODE	ROOTCAUSE
FMEA	TECHNIQUE
HEPARIN	TRAILINGZERO
HIGHALERT	UNAUTHORIZED

Chapter *18*

Durable and Nondurable Medical Equipment, Devices, and Supplies

Learning Outcomes

This chapter reinforces the following learning outcomes discussed in Chapter 18/Durable and Nondurable Medical Equipment, Devices, and Supplies of the *Manual for Pharmacy Technicians, 4th edition*.

- Describe the characteristics of durable and nondurable medical equipment.
- Identify the various types of blood glucose meters and continuous glucose monitoring systems.
- Describe the steps in measuring blood glucose.
- Describe the nondurable medical supplies used in insulin delivery, blood glucose, and lab monitoring.
- Explain the methods of insulin delivery using syringes, continuous infusion pumps, and insulin pens.
- Identify the various types of blood pressure monitors and explain the methods of measuring blood pressure.
- Identify commonly used pedometers and heart rate monitors.
- List the advantages and disadvantages of home diagnostic products and identify commonly used products.
- Identify orthopedic support products.
- Describe the purpose of ostomy products.

Multiple Choice 104

Matching 105

True or False 106

Fill in the Blank 106

Short Answer 106

Word Search 107

Multiple Choice

1. DME stands for:

   a. Drug manufacturer equipment.
   b. Division of medical equipment.
   c. Durable medical equipment.
   d. Devices for medical expenditures.

2. According to the American Diabetes Association, plasma blood glucose levels before meals should be:

   a. 10-60 mg/dL.
   b. 60-80 mg/dL.
   c. 70-130 mg/dL.
   d. 100-180 mg/dL.

3. Blood glucose meters vary in features such as:

   a. The size of blood sample needed for testing.
   b. The need for calibration of the meter.
   c. The testing time and memory of test results.
   d. All of the above.
   e. None of the above.

4. Complications of diabetes include:

   a. An increased risk of heart disease and stroke.
   b. Blindness and kidney failure.
   c. Nerve damage and amputations.
   d. All of the above.
   e. None of the above.

5. Sites for insulin injection include:

   a. The abdomen.
   b. The inner wrist area.
   c. The shoulder.
   d. All of the above.
   e. None of the above.

6. Insulin syringes are available in:

   a. 30-unit (3/10 mL).
   b. 50-unit (0.5 mL).
   c. 100-unit (1 mL).
   d. All of the above.
   e. None of the above.

7. Advantages of insulin pump therapy include the following:

   a. More accurate insulin delivery than injections.
   b. Fewer variations in blood glucose levels and reduction in episodes of low blood sugar and flexibility in mealtimes and physical activity.
   c. Ability to administer additional insulin based upon carbohydrate intake and blood glucose levels.
   d. All of the above.
   e. None of the above.

8. Disadvantages of insulin pump therapy include the following:

   a. Weight loss.
   b. Diabetic ketoacidosis (DKA).
   c. More variations of hemoglobin A1c level.
   d. All of the above.
   e. None of the above.

9. Normal heart rate ranges for adults, 18 years of age or older, are:

   a. 30-70 beats per minute.
   b. 60-100 beats per minute.
   c. 80-120 beats per minute.
   d. 90-140 beats per minute.

10. The home HIV test kits provide results:

   a. That are considered to be 99.9% accurate.
   b. In 7 days after the blood sample arrives at a designated laboratory.
   c. That are retrieved by calling a toll-free number.
   d. All of the above.
   e. None of the above.

Matching

Matching I
Match the insulins below to the correct duration of action.

A. Rapid-Acting

B. Short-Acting

C. Intermediate-Acting

D. Long-Acting

_____ 1. Insulin detemir (Levemir)

_____ 2. Insulin lispro (Humalog)

_____ 3. Regular Human (Humulin R, Novolin R)

_____ 4. Insulin glulisine (Apidra)

_____ 5. Insulin aspart (Novolog)

_____ 6. NPH (Humulin N, Novolin N)

_____ 7. Insulin glargine (Lantus)

Part
4

Matching II
Indicate whether the supplies and equipment would be considered Durable Medical Equipment or Nondurable Medical Equipment by placing an A or a B in the space before the numbered items below.

A. Durable Medical Equipment

B. Nondurable Medical Equipment

_____ 1. Absorbent bed pads

_____ 2. Blood glucose meters

_____ 3. Blood glucose test strips and lancets

_____ 4. Blood pressure monitors

_____ 5. Braces

_____ 6. Canes

_____ 7. Commode and shower chairs

_____ 8. Crutches

_____ 9. Diapers

_____ 10. Dressing materials (bandages, gauze dressings, tape)

_____ 11. Exam gloves

_____ 12. Home oxygen equipment

_____ 13. Hospital beds

_____ 14. Infusion pumps

_____ 15. Insulin syringes and pen needles

_____ 16. Nebulizers

_____ 17. Ostomy supplies

_____ 18. Scooters

_____ 19. Suction pumps

_____ 20. Walkers

_____ 21. Wheelchairs

True or False

_____ 1. Any pharmacy that obtains the correct Medicare Part B Forms may bill Medicare for medical equipment.

_____ 2. Hyperglycemia (high blood glucose) and hypoglycemia (low blood glucose) can be identified with the use of insulin pens.

_____ 3. Insulin is classified according to its action (rapid-acting, short-acting, intermediate acting, or long-acting).

_____ 4. The advantage of insulin pens is that they are disposable.

_____ 5. Most disposable insulin pens contain 3 mL or 3000 units of insulin.

_____ 6. Becton Dickinson pen needles are compatible with all insulin pens sold in the United States.

_____ 7. The expiration date of insulin contained in a cartridge or pen can range from 10-42 days.

_____ 8. Since needles are removed after each use, it is acceptable to use an insulin pen in more than one person.

_____ 9. Federal regulations determine the disposal of used needles in home settings.

_____ 10. Hypotension (high blood pressure) is a major risk factor for heart disease, stroke, congestive heart failure, and kidney disease.

_____ 11. A 10% decrease in total blood cholesterol levels can reduce the incidence of heart disease by as much as 30%.

Fill in the Blank

1. A _____ _____ used in blood glucose monitoring contains a reagent that interacts with a blood sample to generate a blood glucose measurement.

2. A _____ (small needle) is used for one-time use to puncture the skin to obtain a blood sample.

3. _____ is a hormone that is produced in the pancreas, which promotes the utilization of glucose, synthesis of protein, and the formation and storage of lipids (fat).

4. Insulin is injected _____ (under the skin).

5. _____ solution is a type of solution that mimics blood and that is used to test the accuracy of a blood glucose meter and test strips.

6. A _____ is a device that records each step a person takes by detecting the motion of the hips.

7. A _____ test gives individuals information about their average blood glucose control for the past 2–3 months in order to determine how well their diabetes treatment plan is working.

8. The best time for fertilization of the egg to occur is within _____ to _____ hours after ovulation.

9. A(n) _____ is a surgically created opening in the body.

10. A(n) _____ is a procedure that diverts urine from the bladder.

Short Answer

1. Describe the steps for monitoring blood glucose.

2. Describe the steps for an insulin injection.

3. Describe the process for monitoring blood pressure.

4. Explain how the various types of pedometers work.

5. Discuss the failures of home pregnancy tests.

Word Search

```
I M S U B C U T A N E O U S Y B A R U D L O S O A
L H E E I N S U L I N I N F U S I O N O D O U I O
N O E S U F N I N I L U S N I R I B O L G O M E H
O S O M E D M O N I E E B L O E A B S O O R S S S
R D I S O T L Y I B N L N E E T N B P E O A O E E
I P N N I G M B O P C B U M I E E L I O E O R E T
O L E O L O L L A R E A Y P T M R O R L M N E E U
E L E M T O G O D R T R T I O O O O T C T R M N S
B B D S O O M L B D U U Y U H D I D S O U L E A E
E B O A M I B A H I T D D Q T E D P T S S R R T C
D L R E O A A R O A N M N E R P S R S O T M U U N
E O H I R I M O N I T O R O O O U E E L D S S C R
R O H U R O R T H O T I C R N E R S T E I A S B U
C D D S U B C U T A N E N T E P G S O R I C E U A
C G A N E R O S P L Y N E H D R S U E O I I R S S
O L O O S I N S O M O O U O O O S O T T B U D T E
U U I Y M O T S O R U B O P U M A T O T T E O P C
I C U A C E T T I P S L U E O I O H O E E E O E S
O O M E H O S I O L B T N D E S R R Y O C E L D H
I S N O I O V I C S H E E I N O O L U L N C B O E
S E R I L E O S T O M Y N C A H T T O I A O E M P
U M E O B T A L A N C E U D T C E I N B L L O I R
F E C L A I C N L C P D R E U B R M O M B U C T O
N T O U R S L S U N I T T V C E V L O A B E E O L
I L R F U O E O E O C B S I B C Q P R G T R U R L
N L L E D O T L R L E T O C U O P U O T L C C T T
I C A O N S U I B R C U T E S U D E I O U A E U T
L T A T O S N T U E C U U S R N E S D P H M B T B
U E C E N A S T O M Y P D B O O U I O O M N U I B
S C L I T E U I N S U L I N P E F L O M M E S C N
N I U U B I N E P N I L U S N I U O E I L E N R R
I R E T E M E S O C U L G D O O L B B L N U M T U
I Y M O T S O L A C D U I L C V T N I M P U I Q E
T E S T S T R I I I S L P M O N I T E R I C T O T
A R O U O S T O M Y I L O E S T O M Y M R C R Y I
E S N T L A B E E C B A O M I R N L D A C S O O S
```

ANEROID

BLOODGLUCOSEMETER

BLOODPRESSURE

CLIA

COLOSTOMY

DURABLE

EQUIPMENT

HEMOGLOBIN

ILEOSTOMY

INSULININFUSION

INSULINPEN

LANCET

MONITOR

NONDURABLE

ORTHOPEDICDEVICES

ORTHOTIC

OSTOMY

PEDOMETER

SUBCUTANEOUS

TESTSTRIPS

UROSTOMY

Chapter 19

Purchasing and Inventory Control

Learning Outcomes

This chapter reinforces the following learning outcomes discussed in Chapter 19/ Purchasing and Inventory Control of the *Manual for Pharmacy Technicians, 4th edition*.

- Demonstrate an understanding of the formulary system and its application in a purchasing and inventory system.
- Execute lending and borrowing pharmaceutical transactions between pharmacies.
- Apply the proper principles and processes when receiving and storing pharmaceuticals.
- Identify key techniques for reviewing packaging, labeling, and storage considerations when handling pharmaceutical products.
- Demonstrate an understanding of pharmaceutical products that require special handling within the purchasing and inventory system.
- Demonstrate both an understanding and the application of appropriate processes for maintaining and managing a pharmaceutical inventory.
- Complete the appropriate processes in the handling of pharmaceutical recalls and the disposal of pharmaceutical products.

Multiple Choice 110

Matching 111

True or False 112

Fill in the Blank 113

Short Answer 113

Alphabet Soup 113

Multiple Choice

1. With regard to the National Drug Code, the first set of digits identifies the:

   a. Package type and size.
   b. Specific drug manufacturer or labeler of the product.
   c. Product code, denoting the formulation, dosage form, and strength.
   d. None of the above.

2. A hospital P&T Committee is generally comprised of:

   a. Nurses, pharmacists and risk managers.
   b. Administrators, purchasing agents, and pharmacists.
   c. Physicians, pharmacists, nurses, and administrators.
   d. Pharmacists, pharmacy technicians, and purchasing agents.

3. The members of the P&T Committee collaborate to choose medications for the formulary that are the:

   a. Safest.
   b. Most effective.
   c. Least costly.
   d. All of the above.
   e. None of the above.

4. A hospital formulary is generally formatted to inform users of:

   a. Product availability.
   b. The appropriate therapeutic uses of medications.
   c. Recommended dosing and administration of medications.
   d. All of the above.
   e. None of the above.

5. An advantage of a wholesaler arrangement is that wholesalers:

   a. Agree to deliver 95 to 98% of the items on schedule and offer a 24-hour/7-day-per-week emergency service.
   b. Provide the pharmacy with electronic order entry/receiving devices, a computer system for ordering, bar coded shelf stickers, and a printer for order confirmation printouts.
   c. Offer a highly competitive discount (minus 1 to 2%) below product cost/contract pricing and competitive alternate contract pricing.
   d. All of the above.
   e. None of the above.

6. Technicians should pay close attention to these three main issues of product similarity:

   a. Similar tablet color, therapeutic class, manufacturer.
   b. Similar package inserts, expiration dates, control schedules.
   c. Similar drug names, package sizes, label format.
   d. Similar capsule sizes, cap colors, costs.

7. Traditional inventory management and handling practices do not work well with medication samples because:

   a. Medication samples are not ordered or dispensed by the pharmacy.
   b. Samples are provided to physicians on request by the drug manufacturer and are free of charge.
   c. Samples may not be medications on the formulary.
   d. All of the above.
   e. None of the above.

8. The most common reason that drugs are returned to the manufacturer is because they:

   a. Expired.
   b. Were ordered in error.
   c. Were damaged in shipment.
   d. Were shipped in error.

9. A report following a multiple-month study of environmental impact of pharmaceutical waste indicates that trace amounts of pharmaceuticals are present in the drinking water of 24 major U.S. metropolitan cities nationwide due to:

   a. Human excretion.
   b. The routine waste disposal of medication by consumers.
   c. The routine waste disposal of medication by pharmacies.
   d. All of the above.
   e. None of the above.

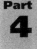

10. Recalls initiated by manufacturers and distributors:

    a. Are more efficient and effective in ensuring timely consumer protection than an FDA-initiated court action or seizure of the product.

    b. Are phoned to pharmacies by the manufacturer of the product or by drug wholesalers.

    c. Include a phone number for pharmacies to call to find out the class of recall, the reason for recall, the name of the recalled product, the manufacturer, all affected lot numbers of the product, and response required.

    d. Typically do not include instructions on the extent of action required in contacting affected patients.

Matching

Match the following actual recalls with the correct class used for their recalls. Hint: There are four recalls in each class.

A. Class I: The most serious of recalls; ongoing product use may result in serious health threat or death.

B. Class II: Moderate severity concern; ongoing product use may pose serious adverse events or irreversible consequences.

C. Class III: Lowest severity concern; ongoing product use unlikely to cause adverse health threat; however, a marginal chance of injury may exist, so the product is being recalled.

_____ 1. PRODUCT M.V.I. ADULT (Multi-Vitamin Infusion), 10 mL UNIT VIAL

REASON: Subpotent (Multiple Ingredient Drug): The discolored top chamber solution does not meet the visual appearance specification. This discoloration potentially impacts the potency of the Biotin and Folic Acid contained in the top chamber.

_____ 2. PRODUCT Fentanyl Transdermal System 75 mcg/hr, 5 systems per box

REASON: Incorrect NDC bar code label on the outer carton; bar code is indicated for the 100 mcg/hr strength instead of the 75 mcg/hr strength. The immediate package label is correct.

_____ 3. PRODUCT ALLOPURINOL Tablets, USP, 100 mg, 30 Tablets

REASON: Labeling: Correct Labeled Product Mispack; 100 mg bottles packed in shipping boxes labeled as 300 mg.

_____ 4. PRODUCT Propofol Injectable Emulsion 1%, 200 mg/20 mL, (10 mg/mL), 20 ml vials

REASON: Lack of Sterility Assurance: The product was manufactured on equipment found to be contaminated with microbiological organisms.

_____ 5. PRODUCT Isosorbide Mononitrate, 60 mg

REASON: The products may contain oversized tablets.

_____ 6. PRODUCT NIKKI HASKELL'S StarCaps Diet System Dietary Supplement Capsules

REASON: Unapproved new drug; the dietary supplement lots contain the undeclared drug ingredient Bumetanide, a prescription diuretic.

_____ 7. PRODUCT Liothyronine Sodium Tablets, USP 5 mcg

REASON: The recall is being conducted due to a stability failure at the 12-month time point; the assay value of this lot was found to be subpotent.

_____ 8. PRODUCT IBUDONE (hydrocodone bitartrate and ibuprofen tablets), 5 mg/200 mg

REASON: Subpotent (Multiple Ingredient Drug): Below specification for the assay at the room temperature 3-month stability time-point for Ibuprofen and Hydrocodone Bitartrate.

_____ 9. PRODUCT 1) Honey Lemon Soothing Cough Drops (Menthol) 9.1 mg, Individually twist wrapped drops

REASON: Subpotent (Single Ingredient Drug): Cough drops are out of specification for menthol.

_____ 10. PRODUCT Ondansetron in 5% Dextrose Injection, 32 mg/50 mL (0.64 mg/mL), Single-Dose Premix Bag

REASON: Non-Sterility: This product is being recalled because a white feathery substance found floating inside the IV bag was identified as mold.

_____ 11. RIPPED TABS TR tablets, Anabolic Amplifier Proprietary Blend

REASON: Marketed Without an Approved NDA/ANDA: 62 products marketed as dietary supplements have been found to contain steroid or steroid-like substances, making them unapproved new drugs.

_____ 12. PRODUCT Sertraline Tablets, 50 mg bottles of 90

REASON: Incorrect medication guides shipped with product.

True or False

_____ 1. A hospital formulary is developed and maintained by a committee of medical and allied health staff called the Pharmacy and Therapeutics (P&T) Committee.

_____ 2. Formularies are not a concern in retail pharmacy.

_____ 3. When there is a request for use of products that are not on the official hospital formulary, the pharmacist must refuse the request and offer a comparable or therapeutically equivalent product.

_____ 4. Independent community pharmacies typically do not become members of a GPO.

_____ 5. Purchasing contracts can involve sole-source or multisource products. Sole-source branded products are available from only one manufacturer, whereas multisource generic products are available from numerous manufacturers.

_____ 6. A GPO guarantees the price of pharmaceuticals over the established contract period, which is usually 3-6 months.

_____ 7. It is important that the pharmacy technician documents any off-contract purchases resulting from manufacturers' inability to supply a given product that the pharmacy is buying on contract, which may require the pharmacy to buy or substitute a competing product that is not on contract at a higher cost.

_____ 8. For most pharmacies, the advantages of direct ordering outweigh the disadvantages.

_____ 9. Some drugs can only be purchased directly from the manufacturers.

_____ 10. Borrowing or lending drugs between pharmacies is not allowed due to federal restrictions.

_____ 11. In a reliable and efficient receiving system, the personnel responsible for ordering should be the same as the receiving personnel.

_____ 12. Just as checking the product label carefully is important when a prescription or medication order is filled, taking the same care when receiving pharmaceuticals and accurately placing them in their storage location are essential for prevention of medication errors.

_____ 13. Research on tall man lettering has failed to demonstrate effectiveness in distinguishing similarities and preventing look-alike, sound-alike drug mix-ups.

_____ 14. If a hospital uses a BCMA system, it is critical that each bar code on items new to the facility be scanned at the time that each product is received to ensure that the product bar code is in the BCMA system. This does not apply to products that have been received before from the same manufacturer.

_____ 15. Schedule III, IV, and V controlled substances are generally obtained in a manner identical to that for Schedule II substances.

_____ 16. The difficult logistical and control factors of medication samples have led many organizations to adopt policies that simply disallow medication samples.

Fill in the Blank

1. There is an FDA database that utilizes a unique identification number, called the _____ _____ _____, to identify drug products that are intended for human consumption or use.

2. Most hospitals and health care systems develop a list of medications that may be prescribed for patients in the institution or health care system, called a _____.

3. Most health system pharmacies are members of a _____ _____ _____, which contracts with manufacturers to purchase pharmaceuticals at discounted prices, in return for a guaranteed minimum purchase volume.

4. _____ purchasing from a manufacturer involves the execution of a purchase order (PO) from the pharmacy to the manufacturer of the drug.

5. The _____ (also known as distributor) usually operates a large-scale warehouse in various geographic regions and exists to help bring pharmaceutical products closer to the market.

6. When a health system pharmacy agrees to purchase most (e.g., 90 to 95%) of its pharmaceuticals from a single wholesale company, a _____ vendor arrangement is established, and, customarily, a contract between the pharmacy and the drug wholesaler is developed.

7. The process of receiving medications and putting them in their proper location, and placing products that will expire in the near future in the front of the shelf or bin, and the newly acquired products (with longer shelf lives) behind packages that will expire before them is a common practice known as _____ _____.

8. The convention of labeling pharmaceuticals with mixed case labeling also known as _____ _____ _____ is an important tactic employed in the interest of calling attention to similarities in drug names. Research on this approach has demonstrated effectiveness in distinguishing similarities and preventing look-alike, sound-alike drug mix-ups.

9. When an order is received and checked in, the products' expiration dates should be checked to ensure that it meets the department's minimum expiration date requirement. Frequently, departments require that products received have a minimum shelf life of _____ _____ remaining before they expire.

10. When controlled substances are inventoried and tracked continuously, this type of inventory method is referred to as a _____ inventory process.

11. Regulations specific to Schedule II controlled substances require DEA form _____ to be completed to initiate procurement of these products.

12. A simple means of calculating total inventory _____ in a given period is to divide the total purchases in that period by the value of physical inventory taken at a reasonable single point in time.

Short Answer

1. Describe the receiving process and explain the financial implications.

2. Discuss the special processes required for ordering, receiving, and storing controlled substances. Where would you look to find more information?

3. Explain the considerations when receiving and storing chemotherapeutic medications.

4. Investigational drugs require special record-keeping. Discuss the types of records that need to be kept for investigational drugs.

5. What does RDDS stand for? Discuss the purpose and give examples.

Alphabet Soup

There are many acronyms used in the medical profession. Fill in the full name of each acronym below.

a. PO

b. GPO

c. FDA

d. NDC

e. DRLS

f. AWP

g. PBM

h. BCMA

i. DEA

j. IRB

k. RDDS

l. MSDS

m. DOT

n. RCRA

o. EPA

p. GMP

q. NDA

r. ANDA

s. IMPACT

t. WHO

Part

4

Chapter 20

Billing and Reimbursement

Learning Outcomes

This chapter reinforces the following learning outcomes discussed in Chapter 20/ Billing and Reimbursement of the *Manual for Pharmacy Technicians, 4th edition.*

- Explain the basic principles of pharmacy billing and reimbursement.
- Define common pricing benchmarks.
- Describe the differences in reimbursement processes dependent on pharmaceuticals and pharmacy services.
- Describe the categories of information that are needed to submit a third-party claim for a prescription or medication order.
- Use knowledge of third-party insurance billing procedures to identify a reason for a rejected claim.

Multiple Choice 116

Matching 117

True or False 118

Fill in the Blank 118

Short Answer 118

Crossword Puzzle 119

Multiple Choice

1. The exact methodology that is used to bill and reimburse for drugs varies based on several factors, including the following:

   a. The practice setting in which the drug is dispensed.
   b. The type of drug that is being dispensed (e.g., single-source brand products vs. multisource generic products).
   c. The party who is paying for the drugs.
   d. All of the above.
   e. None of the above.

2. Overhead costs often include various expenses such as:

   a. Rent and utilities.
   b. Personnel costs (i.e., salaries for pharmacists and technicians).
   c. Equipment (computers, fax, printer).
   d. Supplies (labels, vials, etc.).
   e. All of the above.
   f. None of the above.

3. In community pharmacy practice, the most common type of payment method is:

   a. Prospective.
   b. Retrospective.

4. The most common purchasers of private insurance are:

   a. Employers and labor unions.
   b. Trust funds.
   c. Professional associations.
   d. All of the above.
   e. None of the above.

5. PBMs and their sponsors:

   a. Develop formularies and negotiate discounts or rebates with pharmaceutical companies.
   b. Track patient allergies.
   c. Keep track of all prescriptions dispensed and sent to employers.
   d. All of the above.
   e. None of the above.

6. Medicare is the federal health program for:

   a. The elderly and the disabled.
   b. People with end-stage renal disease.
   c. People with amyotrophic lateral sclerosis (ALS).
   d. All of the above.
   e. None of the above.

7. Medicare Part B pays for:

   a. Medically necessary services.
   b. Medically necessary supplies.
   c. Some preventative services.
   d. All of the above.
   e. None of the above.

8. Individuals with Part B coverage are responsible for the:

   a. Premium.
   b. Deductible.
   c. Copayment.
   d. All of the above.
   e. None of the above.

9. Part A coverage is:

   a. Pre-paid through payroll taxes.
   b. Optional medical insurance for outpatient physician and hospital services, clinical laboratory services, and durable medical equipment, prosthetics, orthotics, and supplies.
   c. The Medicare Advantage Plan, which combines Part B and C coverage.
   d. A federal prescription drug program that is paid for by the Centers for Medicare and Medicaid Services (CMS).

10. During the coverage gap, the beneficiary:

    a. Pays no costs for prescriptions.
    b. Pays 10% of the cost of prescriptions.
    c. Pays 75% of the cost of prescriptions.
    d. Must pay all costs for prescriptions.

Matching

Match the correct Medicare plan with its name.

Part A

Part B

Part C

Part D

_____ 1. Prescription drug coverage

_____ 2. Hospital insurance

_____ 3. Medical insurance

_____ 4. Medicare Advantage plans

Match the listed DAW codes (0-9) with the correct description

0

1

2

3

4

5

6

7

8

9

_____ 5. Brand-Name Drug Mandated by Law: substitution not allowed

_____ 6. Brand Name Dispensed at Generic Price: substitution allowed

_____ 7. Override

_____ 8. Generic not in stock: substitution allowed

_____ 9. Patient DAW: substitution allowed; patient requested product dispensed

_____ 10. Physician DAW: substitution not allowed by provider

_____ 11. Generic or Single-Source Brand: no product selection

_____ 12. Other

_____ 13. Pharmacist-Selected Brand Name: substitution allowed; pharmacist-selected product

_____ 14. Generic not available: substitution allowed

True or False

_____ 1. Typically, the reimbursement formula for a generic product is the same as that for a brand product.

_____ 2. Some third-party payers may pay a higher dispensing fee for generic drugs or formulary products as an incentive to encourage utilization of preferred products.

_____ 3. In the IPAP model, pharmacies typically receive payment for medications that have already been dispensed.

_____ 4. Medicare Part B, which covers outpatient physician and hospital services, clinical laboratory services, and durable medical equipment, prosthetics, orthotics, and supplies (DMEPOS), is automatic medical insurance for those 65 and older.

_____ 5. Medicare Part D is a federal prescription drug program that is paid for by the Centers for Medicare and Medicaid Services (CMS) and by individual premiums.

_____ 6. Since drug formularies for Medicare Part D vary from plan to plan, beneficiaries must be careful when choosing a Medicare prescription drug plan to ensure that their prescription drugs are covered.

_____ 7. CMS requires that all Medicare prescription drug plans cover at least six drugs in each of the ten therapeutic categories.

_____ 8. If a beneficiary has a prescription for a drug that requires prior authorization from the Part D plan, the prescribing physician needs to obtain prior authorization for the drug before the claim can be paid.

_____ 9. All Part D claims must contain a National Provider Identifier (NPI) for the prescriber, or may substitute the provider's DEA number.

_____ 10. Medicaid is another term for Medicare.

_____ 11. As of April 1, 2008, all Medicaid prescriptions must be electronically prescribed or written/printed on "tamper resistant" paper.

_____ 12. By law, Medicaid recipients may not be denied services based on their inability to pay the assigned cost sharing.

Fill in the Blank

1. In simple accounting terms, _____ represents the inflow of funds.

2. _____ payment typically includes all costs associated with treating a particular condition, including medications and pharmacies challenged to deliver drugs at or below the predetermined rate in order to ensure that drug costs are covered.

3. Insurance companies or pharmacy benefit managers are considered _____ payers.

4. The _____ is the cost-sharing amount paid by the patient or customer.

5. _____ was created in the 1960s and was the first generally accepted standard pricing benchmark.

6. Many drug companies offer certain free drugs through _____ _____ _____ to low-income patients who lack prescription drug coverage and meet certain criteria.

7. _____ _____ _____ are organizations that administer pharmacy benefits for private or public third-party payers, also known as plan sponsors.

8. The _____ is the cornerstone of any PBM activities. It is a specific list of drugs that is included with a given pharmacy benefit.

9. For Part A claims, _____ _____ is the basis for reimbursement.

10. Medicaid recipients who also qualify for Medicare are known as _____ _____.

Short Answer

1. Explain step therapy.

2. Discuss the steps in processing third-party prescriptions, possible rejections that may occur, and possible solutions to the rejections.

3. Explain the difference between prospective and retrospective payment.

4. Discuss the programs available for those without insurance.

Crossword Puzzle

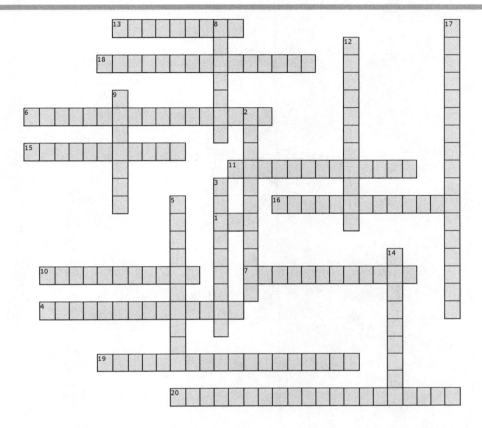

Across:

1. A set rate paid for an inpatient procedure based on cost and intensity. Drugs provided during an inpatient stay are not separately reimbursed; they are included in the DRG payment

4. Set upper limits of an amount of a drug that is covered by the benefit, or the total days of therapy

6. Price based on manufacturer-reported selling price data and includes volume discounts and price concessions that are offered to all classes of trade

7. Determination of the insurer's payment after the member's insurance benefits are applied to a medical claim

10. A percentage charge for a service such as a prescription or doctor visit

11. A method of payment in which providers bill separately for each patient encounter or service they provide

13. An amount that insured individuals must pay for a service, such as a prescription or doctor visit, each time they use the insurance benefit

15. Requiring the use of a recognized first-line drug before a more complex or expensive second-line drug is used

16. The amount paid for dispensing the prescription

18. An organization (either private or public) that reimburses a pharmacy or patient for products and/or services

19. The amount to be paid for drugs is predetermined based on the condition that is being treated

20. Drugs are dispensed and reimbursed later, according to a predetermined formula that is specified in a contract between the pharmacy and the third-party payer

Down:

2. Also referred to as the "donut hole"

3. A system of health insurance in which the insurer pays for the cost of covered services after care has been given on a fee-for-service basis. It usually defines the maximum amounts covered

5. A fixed amount that must be paid each year by the individual before the insurance starts to pay

8. A group of pharmacies, physicians, hospitals, or other providers who participate in a certain managed care plan

9. Represents the inflow of funds

12. The amount of insurance costs shared by the employee or beneficiary

14. A specific list of drugs that are included with a given prescription drug plan

17. The maximum of federal matching funds that the federal government will pay to state Medicaid programs for eligible generic and multisource drugs

Answer Key

Chapter 1 Key 122

Chapter 2 Key 126

Chapter 3 Key 129

Chapter 4 Key 133

Chapter 5 Key 136

Chapter 6 Key 139

Chapter 7 Key 142

Chapter 8 Key 148

Chapter 9 Key 150

Chapter 10 Key 153

Chapter 11 Key 157

Chapter 12 Key 160

Chapter 13 Key 165

Chapter 14 Key 168

Chapter 15 Key 170

Chapter 16 Key 174

Chapter 17 Key 178

Chapter 18 Key 182

Chapter 19 Key 185

Chapter 20 Key 190

Chapter 1 Answer Keys

Multiple Choice Key

1. d. Advising patients about aspirin. *Technicians are not allowed to offer any type of clinical advice.*

2. d. Pharmacy Technician certificate. *PTCB provides a national certification exam, as does ICPT.*

3. a. Provision of a separate credential to be used after the technician's name. *Accredited programs must include standard learning objectives so that technician education is current, standard, and complete. Pharmacy technicians who complete accredited pharmacy technician education will receive a certificate of completion from ASHP. However, they are not provided with a separate credential to be used after their name.*

4. d. Ambulatory pharmacy. *Pharmacy technicians have the most patient contact with customers in pharmacies where customers walk in to obtain their prescriptions.*

5. b. PBM stands for *pharmacy benefit manager.*

6. a. Medication therapy management (MTM) includes all of the following except assessment of a pharmacy's inventory. *Inventory is a nonclinical task so it would not be part of MTM.*

7. b. Pharmaceutical care includes all of the following except compounding sterile medications using aseptic technique. *Compounding sterile medications using aseptic technique is a physical task rather than a clinical task.*

8. b. Pharmacokinetics is the study of the process by which drugs are absorbed, distributed, metabolized, and eliminated in the body. *Pharmacokinetics is the movement (kinesis) of medications through the body from absorption to elimination.*

9. b. In all states, pharmacists must be licensed by the State Board of Pharmacy. *Each state has its own State Board of Pharmacy, which is charged with protecting the public. One way boards do this is by setting the criteria for licensure of pharmacists.*

10. d. ASHP's ten characteristics of a professional include all of the following except ability to defend medication errors. *Professionals must be knowledgeable and possess skills of the profession, be committed to self-improvement of skills and knowledge, and must be accountable for their work. Medical errors must be handled diligently rather than "defended."*

11. d. Technician duties in a home care setting may include all of the following except discussing drug interactions. *Discussion of drug interactions is a clinical function requiring a pharmacist's clinical judgment.*

12. a. As the demand for cost-effective health care increases, pharmacy technicians with well-developed critical thinking skills may find themselves assuming responsibilities previously assigned to pharmacists such as managerial duties. *Management is an area of pharmacy where technicians may be of great assistance.*

Matching Key

1. C
2. D
3. A
4. B
5. F
6. H
7. J
8. G
9. E
10. I

True or False Answer Key

1. True. The study of how drugs are absorbed, distributed, metabolized, and eliminated by the body is called pharmacokinetics.

2. False. Educating patients about their medications or suggesting medication alternatives to physicians is a task for a pharmacy technician. *Only pharmacists can educate patients about their medications because this task requires professional clinical judgment.*

3. False. Training prerequisites for pharmacy technicians are the same throughout all of the states. *Currently, each state may determine the requirements for pharmacy technicians.*

4. False. Only pharmacists may prepare and compound sterile products. *Pharmacists must check all work, but pharmacy technicians often prepare and compound sterile products.*

5. True. Technicians may be trained on the job or by completing a formal program. *Depending on states requirements, either of these options may be used currently for technician training.*

6. False. Pharmacists may be trained on the job or by completing a formal program. *Currently, pharmacists must earn a PharmD degree and pass a test. Older pharmacists may have a BS degree instead of a PharmD degree and have passed a test.*

7. True. Pharmacy technicians must recertify every 2 years by completing 20 hours of continuing education, with at least 1 hour related to pharmacy law.

8. False. Pharmacy technician training programs are accredited by PTCB. *Pharmacy technician training programs are accredited by ASHP.*

9. False. Residencies provide the opportunity for pharmacy technicians to gain clinical experience, usually in hospital, ambulatory, or community settings. *Residencies are opportunities for pharmacists.*

10. True. Most consumers believe that all pharmacy technicians have been trained and certified before they are allowed to prepare prescriptions.

11. False. There are three recognized certification tests—PTCE, ExCPT, and NPTE. *Only PTCE and ExCPT are recognized certification tests.*

Fill in the Blank Answer Key

1. 20
2. 2
3. 1
4. 90 (10 of these are not scored)
5. 110 (10 of these are not included in the score)
6. 10
7. Hospice or palliative
8. Hospital pharmacy or long-term care
9. Community, retail, home care, or mail order
10. PBM or pharmacy benefit manager

Short Answer Key

1. A pharmacy technician's first consideration is to ensure the health and safety of the patient. This technician's first concern was his lunch. The technician displayed unethical behavior in the form of dishonesty and a lack of integrity by providing inaccurate information. His demonstration of incompetence in his position discredits the profession and reflects poorly upon the employer.

2. Technicians in community settings often prepare prescription labels for checking by a pharmacist, order and maintain drug inventory, process insurance claims, and operate a cash register. In some states, pharmacy technicians may fill prescriptions to be checked later by a pharmacist.

Pharmacy technicians in hospitals may enter physician medication orders into the pharmacy computer system, prepare IV drug admixtures, repackage and label unit dose medications, restock automated dispensing cabinets, deliver medications, and complete paperwork for quality assurance or billing purposes. In some hospitals, pharmacy technicians may dispense medications from a preapproved list or even administer some types of medications.

In both settings, good communication skills, including telephone etiquette and the ability to interpret nonverbal body language, are critical for technicians because they have a lot of interaction with other staff in hospitals and with staff and the public in community settings. Pharmacy technicians must be familiar with brand and generic names, dosage forms, and therapeutic uses of common prescription and over-the-counter medications in both settings.

3. Medication Therapy Management (MTM) has become the pharmacy practice model. In 2003, the Medicare Modernization Act was signed into federal law. Under this act, Medicare prescription drug providers are required to establish MTM programs that improve medication use and reduce adverse events. Medication therapy management has been defined as "a distinct service or group of services that optimize therapeutic outcomes for individual patients. Medication therapy management services are independent of, but can occur in conjunction with, the provision of a medication product. These services include assessment of a patient's health status; formulation of a medication treatment plan; selection, initiation, modification, or administration of medication therapy; monitoring of the patient's response to therapy; review of medications for medication-related problems; documentation and communication of care; provision of patient education and information to increase patient understanding and appropriate use of medications; and coordination and integration of MTM services into the broader health care services provided to the patient."

4.

	PTCB	ICPT
Established	1995	2005
Web address	www.ptcb.org	http://www.national techexam.org/excptinfo .html
Test time	Two-hour test	Two-hour test
Test description	Eighty multiple-choice questions plus an additional ten non-scored questions	110 multiple-choice questions (10 of these are not counted in the score)

5. ASHP

6. Inventory purchasing and management—This position is commonly seen in hospital pharmacies. It is usually a Monday through Friday job, and requires skills in spreadsheets and contracts as well as attention to detail.

Sterile product preparation—Work in a clean room is a highly popular specialty for technicians because it is often fast paced and requires dexterity and math skills.

Surgical pharmacy—In larger hospitals, there are satellite pharmacies to provide support to surgery suites. This may include some sterile preparation of medications as well as maintenance of anesthesia carts, perfusion kits, trauma kits, and other specialized medications depending on the types of surgeries commonly performed.

Nuclear pharmacy—This area of pharmacy requires education beyond initial technician training. It is a very specialized field, and a nuclear pharmacy may serve a large geographical area.

Veterinary pharmacy—This specialty may involve preparation of sterile products as well as extemporaneous compounding also known as nonsterile compounding in order to prepare unique doses of medications (large for elephants or small for mice). Variety is a key attraction in most cases.

Internet Research Key

1. a. The PTCE applies to all practice settings. In preparing for the PTCE, familiarity with the material contained in basic pharmacy technician training manuals or books may be helpful. Your supervising pharmacist may also be helpful in designing a study plan. The PTCB does not endorse or sponsor any review course, manuals, or books for the PTCB exam. A full content online is available through the links listed on the right side of this page.

   b. The exam is made of three basic knowledge functions:

      I. Assisting the Pharmacist in Serving Patients
      II. Maintaining Medication and Inventory Control Systems
      III. Participating in the Administration and Management of Pharmacy Practice

   c. The PTCE contains 90 multiple-choice questions. Ten of the 90 questions are pre-test questions and will not count toward your final score. The pre-test questions provide statistical information for possible use on future examinations; this information is vital in building a quality test.

   d. Candidates will have 2 hours to complete the exam tutorial, the PTCE, and exit survey.

2. a. As a pharmacy technician, you are a vital part of the health-system pharmacy team. ASHP helps you prepare for an increasingly responsible role in the pharmacy department and develop your full professional potential with a host of technician-focused CE, educational programming, resources, and member services.

   b. The Pharmacy Technician Initiative is a partnership between ASHP and individual state affiliates to advocate for state laws that require, as a prerequisite for state board registration, completion of an ASHP-accredited pharmacy technician training and Pharmacy Technician Certification Board (PTCB) certification.

3. a. Newsletters can be found at http://www.nabp.net/publications/state-newsletters/

   For Montana, there is a list of proposed changes to several rules as well as an FDA Alert regarding administration of oral nimodipine capsules. There is also an ISMP article called "Safeguards to Implement with 'High Alert' Medications."

   b. Results for "technician" will vary depending on the date you complete this exercise. Here is a sample of what you might find:

   Texas Board Approves PTCB as Single Provider of Technician Certification Exam

   North Carolina News: Item 2207 - Drug Donation Rule Now Effective; Advanced Training Technician Rule Still Pending

   PTCB Certification Required for Technicians by Department of Veterans Affairs

   Continued Efforts to Standardize Pharmacy Technician Education and Training Programs (Resolution No. 106-7-10)

   c. NABP's initiatives are based on the input of its member boards of pharmacy. Each year, NABP members come together to vote on resolutions that ultimately guide the direction of the Association. Recent resolutions addressed the topic of:

   Pharmacy Technician Education Standards

Crossword Puzzle Key

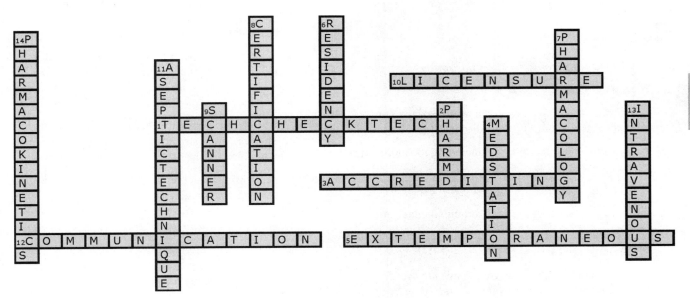

Word Search Key

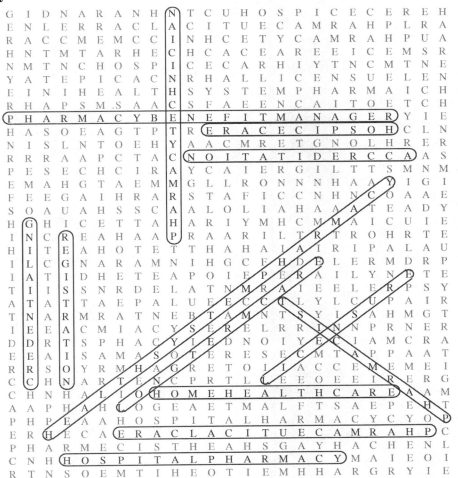

Chapter 2 Answer Keys

Multiple Choice Key

1. b. DEA. *Drug Enforcement Administration.*

2. b. Every 2 years.

3. a. Information received from pharmacies about controlled substance prescriptions dispensed in the state.

4. d. Both laws must be followed, including the more stringent requirements.

5. e. All of the above.

6. a. Enacted by state legislatures through the legislative process.

7. d. All of the above.

8. c. Are not authorized to counsel. *They may translate counseling but may not provide counseling on their own.*

9. b. Up to 5 times within 6 months.

10. a. As needed within 6 months.

Matching Key

1. E
2. K
3. C
4. D
5. B
6. G
7. I
8. L
9. A
10. J
11. F
12. H

True or False Key

1. False. DEA-registered pharmacies are required by law to take an initial inventory of all controlled substances on hand upon commencing operations or upon changes in ownership, with subsequent inventories conducted twice per year thereafter. *Inventories are required every 2 years.*

2. False. The FDA is the federal agency that administers and enforces federal laws for controlled substances and illegal substances such as narcotics and other dangerous drugs. *The DEA is the correct agency.*

3. False. If state and federal laws or regulations differ, the state law has precedence. *If state and federal laws or regulations differ, both must be followed, including the more stringent requirements, whether federal or state.*

4. True. Pharmacy laws are enacted through the state legislature, and pharmacy rules and regulations are adopted through the State Board of Pharmacy.

5. False. Pharmacy technician ratios refer to the numbers of training hours required for specialty practice. *Pharmacy technician ratios refer to the number of pharmacy technicians that may assist a pharmacist at one time.*

6. True. Patient counseling must be provided by the pharmacist. *Pharmacy technicians are not authorized to counsel patients on their medications.*

7. False. The federal law regulating controlled substances is the Federal Food, Drug, and Cosmetic (FDC) Act of 1938. *The federal law regulating controlled substances is the Controlled Substances Act.*

8. True. An example of a Schedule II (CII) medication (one with high potential for abuse or misuse, high risk of dependence) is methylphenidate (Ritalin).

9. False. The statement, "Caution: Federal law prohibits the transfer of this drug to any person other than the patient for whom it was prescribed," must be placed on all labels of legend drugs. *Federal law requires that pharmacies place a specific caution message on the patient container advising the patient that he or she may not give the controlled substance to any other person. "Legend" refers to prescription medications, which may include controlled and non-controlled medications.*

10. True. Prescription monitoring programs monitor prescribing and dispensing of controlled substances.

11. False. Ephedrine and pseudoephedrine, which are the active ingredients in common cough, cold, and allergy products, are precursor chemicals to cocaine and morphine. *Ephedrine and pseudoephedrine, which are the active ingredients in common cough, cold, and allergy products, are precursor chemicals to methamphetamine and amphetamine.*

12. True. The primary federal law establishing health information privacy is the Health Insurance Portability and Accountability Act (HIPAA).

13. False. Prescription monitoring programs have been implemented in all states. *The majority of states have implemented such programs, but not all states have done so.*

Fill in the Blank Key

1. A B
2. 222
3. V
4. 5 6
5. 2
6. 9
7. FDA
8. Bioequivalent
9. Orange Book
10. The Durham-Humphrey Amendment
11. Package insert
12. 80 90

Short Answer Key

1. Percocet is a C-II narcotic, so no refills are allowed by law, and only the quantity indicated on the prescription (not including refill quantities) may be dispensed. The patient would need to be told this. She could discuss the quantity of medication dispensed at one time with her physician.

2. Lomotil is a C-V medication. Therefore, the number of refills is limited by the physician rather than regulation. However, by regulation, those refills must take place within 6 months of the date the prescription is written. Therefore you would need to contact the patient's physician to request a new prescription in this scenario.

3. Pharmacists may only dispense Schedule II controlled substances pursuant to a written prescription signed by the practitioner, unless an exception applies. One exception is in an emergency, in which case the practitioner may telephone or fax the prescription to the pharmacist for a reasonable emergency supply of medication and then provide the original written signed prescription to the pharmacist within 7 days and indicate that it was authorized for emergency dispensing. Another exception is where federal regulations allow facsimile Schedule II prescriptions for patients residing in long-term care facilities or for hospice patients.

4. A prescription for a controlled substance may only be transferred one time. You would need to contact the physician and request a new prescription.

5. Patient counseling is very important to ensure that patients take their medications correctly so that they are safe and effective. Counseling includes providing patients with information about their medications such as what they are for, when and how much to take, whether to take with food, how to store the medication, and possible side effects.

6. Pseudoephedrine
   Ephedrine

7. In addition to the name, manufacturer, dosage form, and dose of the product, information should include uses for the drug (for pain, for constipation), the recommended dosage (suggested daily dose is 2 tablets, which provide 500mg), how often to use the drug (once daily), who should or should not take the medication (for adults and children over the age of 12), information on side effects (may cause drowsiness), information on precautions for using the drug (do not mix with alcohol), total quantity of drug in the container, and expiration date of product.

8. Sublingual nitroglycerin tablets
   Oral contraceptives (birth control pills)

9. Prescription drug products include a package that is not intended for patients. It provides health care professionals with medical and scientific information about the prescription drug. Pharmacists provide patients with different types of written information for their dispensed prescription drugs. Patients are provided with printed information about their dispensed medication called consumer medicine information or CMI. In addition, the FDA requires pharmacists to provide patients with a patient package insert ("PPI") with the dispensing of certain prescription drugs such as estrogens and oral contraceptives. PPIs are written specifically for patient use; whereas, package inserts are developed for use by physicians and pharmacists.

10. State regulations vary. Remember that National Certification is a process through the PTCB or ICPT. You must renew this certification every 2 years by completing continuing education and by submitting requested information and a fee. Registration and licensure are processes through your State Board of Pharmacy. Some states require that you are certified before you can be registered or licensed.

Alphabet Soup Key

a. HIPAA: Health Insurance Portability and Accountability Act

b. DEA: Drug Enforcement Administration

c. FDA: Food and Drug Administration

d. NDA: New Drug Application

e. ANDA: Abbreviated New Drug Application

f. DAW: Dispense As Written

g. DNS: Do Not Substitute

h. NABP: National Association of Boards of Pharmacy

i. OTC: Over the Counter

j. CMEA: The Combat Methamphetamine Epidemic Act of 2005

k. CMI: Consumer Medicine Information

l. PPI: Patient Package Insert

m. PHI: Protected Health Information

n. NACDS: National Association of Chain Drug Stores

Word Search Key

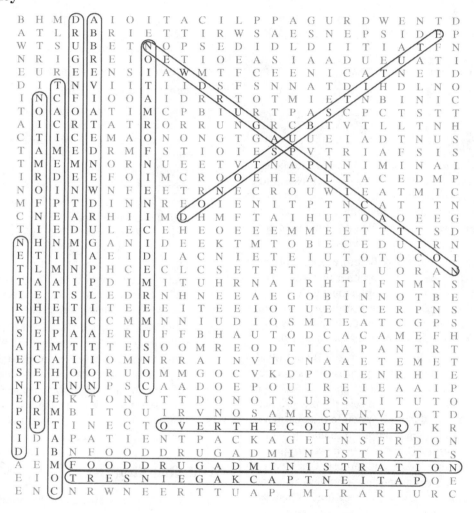

Chapter 3 Answer Keys

Multiple Choice Key

1. c. Adverse drug reaction.
2. c. Only serves patients who walk in or who have medications mailed to them.
3. d. Copayment.
4. c. Medication Guide.
5. a. Durham-Humphrey Amendment.
6. c. Omnibus Budget Reconciliation Act.
7. c. Omnibus Budget Reconciliation Act. When the pharmacists' role changed, it created the need for help in distributive processes of pharmacy.
8. d. Health Insurance Portability and Accountability Act.
9. c. Marital status.
10. d. All of the above.

Matching Key

1. C
2. E
3. A
4. D

True or False Key

1. True. An adverse drug reaction is a bothersome or unwanted effect that results from the use of a drug, unrelated to the intended effect of the drug.

2. False. A generic drug is one that is covered by a patent and is, therefore, only available from a single manufacturer. *A brand drug is covered by a patent.*

3. False. The Health Insurance Portability and Accountability Act (HIPAA) is legislation enacted by states to establish guidelines for the protection of patients' private health information. *HIPAA is a federal law. However, states may also have laws or regulations to protect patients' private health information. If state and federal laws or regulations differ, both must be followed, including the more stringent requirements, whether federal or state.*

4. True. A legend drug is one that, based on safety and potential for addiction, requires authorization from an authorized prescriber before a pharmacist can prepare and dispense the product.

5. True. The foundation of medication therapy management by pharmacists is the proper handling and preparation of the actual drug product by technicians.

6. False. Resolving third-party payer issues is a complicated task usually handled by pharmacists. *Pharmacists depend on skilled technicians to assist with third-party payer issues.*

7. False. If an interaction with a patient seems to be escalating toward confrontation, it is best for the technician to involve another technician. *The technician should involve the pharmacist in this situation.*

8. False. In order to maintain standard workflow, prescriptions should be processed in the order they are received. *It is important for customer service and workflow to ask the patient if he or she will be waiting for the prescription or if he or she will be coming back late, so that prescriptions can be processed in the order in which they are due and when patients expect them to be ready.*

9. True. The use of both isotretinoin and thalidomide is restricted because both medications can cause serious birth defects.

10. True. Counting devices use a scale to count units based on their weight or light beams to count units as they are poured through a machine.

11. False. The only purpose of obtaining patients' signatures is to confirm that they have received the Medication Guides as required by the FDA. *There are three purposes for obtaining patient signatures:*

    1. To document that the patients received a copy of the pharmacy's patient privacy policy in compliance with HIPAA regulations;

    2. To document if the patients refuse patient counseling; and

    3. To document when the patient takes possession of the prescription.

12. True. A pharmacist generally completes special training to become certified to provide disease state management.

Part 1

Fill in the Blank Key

1. Legend or prescription drugs
   Over-the-counter (OTC) drugs

2. Pharmacist

3. Chain

4. Independent

5. FDA

6. REMS

7. Clozapine

8. Copayment or copay

9. Formulary

10. Pharmacy benefit managers (PBMs)

11. Medication Guides

12. NDC number

Short Answer Key

1. There are independent pharmacies owned by one or two people, and chain pharmacies corporately owned. Clinic pharmacies are ambulatory care pharmacies that are located in clinics or medical centers to serve the needs of outpatients. These pharmacies may be owned and operated by the facility, or owned independently but located in the facility. Managed care pharmacies are ambulatory pharmacies that are owned and operated as part of a managed care system such as a health maintenance organization (HMO). Mail-order pharmacies generally fill very large volumes of prescriptions through the mail and specialize in maintenance medications. Because of their high prescription volume, the prescription filling process is often highly automated and there is generally less direct contact with patients, except by telephone and electronically, via web sites and the Internet.

2. When a patient arrives in the pharmacy, correct identification is important. You should check identification with at least two forms of information such as name and date of birth. For a new patient, obtain the correct spelling of the patient name, address and phone number(s), insurance information from patient's insurance card, date of birth, any drug allergies, other prescriptions or OTC medications the patient takes regularly, and significant health conditions. Prescriptions may be received directly from the patient or from the prescriber by telephone, fax, or electronic transmission. Receiving a prescription includes determining whether the prescription will be filled with generic or brand-name drugs. Patients should be informed of their HIPAA rights and should sign a state-ment to that effect. In some pharmacies, the prescription is scanned into the system. The entire filling process for prescriptions is discussed in Chapter 13/Processing Medication Orders and Prescriptions.

3. Prior to OBRA '90, pharmacists spent their time filling prescriptions as ordered by the physician. Pharmacists were not required to keep a patient profile; if one was kept, a review was not required for potential problems with the prescribed drug such as appropriateness of the drug and dose for the patient, drug interactions, or drug duplications. It was not necessary to counsel patients. Since OBRA '90, pharmacists must spend the majority of their time reviewing meds and counseling patients. To augment the pharmacists' time, pharmacy technicians have stepped into the distributive role. Therefore OBRA '90 has added another layer of pharmacy work and created a role for pharmacy technicians.

4. Technicians communicate with patients while ensuring patients' privacy. Technicians receive prescriptions and register patients, enter prescriptions in a computer, handle restricted-use medications, resolve third-party payer issues, fill and label pharmaceutical products, compound prescriptions, collect payment and offer pharmacist-provided patient counseling, and fulfill many miscellaneous responsibilities. Pharmacists must handle all work that requires clinical judgment as well as take responsibility for all technician work. In some states, there are specific instances where technicians may check other technicians' work. This process is called "tech check tech."

5. In addition to making sure you have the correct spelling of a person's name, it is important to be able to contact the patient. Therefore, accurate information such as correct address and phone number(s) are needed. There may be several patients with the same name. In these cases, birth dates may serve as a second identifier for patients. Insurance information from a patient's insurance card will help with processing the prescription. Pharmacists need to know a patient's age, other medications the patient is taking (prescription and OTC), disease states, and drug allergies in order to screen for potential problems with newly prescribed drugs as part of the prospective DUR (drug utilization review) process. Upon review, pharmacists may find problems such as inappropriate drugs for patient age or gender, duplicative therapy, drug interactions, and drug allergies.

6. Alosetron is a drug used to treat severe diarrhea-predominant irritable bowel syndrome (IBS). Due to serious adverse reactions of the gastrointestinal tract, some people necessitate a blood transfusion or surgery and some even lead to death. Alosetron's use is restricted by the Prescription Program for Lotronex (PPL).

The program requires physician enrollment, including submission of the Patient-Physician Agreement Form. Prescriptions must be written by the physician and must include a PPL sticker on the face of the prescription. Refills may be authorized on the prescription.

Clozapine is a drug used to treat patients with schizophrenia. This drug can cause a serious drop in white blood cells, so careful monitoring of these levels must be done regularly based on the patient's condition and medical history. Pharmacies must register to dispense clozapine and only a specific day supply (1, 2, or 3 weeks depending on the patients' monitoring frequency) may be dispensed at a time. The pharmacy must also receive documentation of blood work showing a normal white blood cell count before each dispensing.

Isotretinoin is a drug used for severe acne. Its use is restricted because it can cause serious birth defects. Doctors, patients, and pharmacies must register with the iPledge Program, which monitors the drug's use. Doctors and patients must meet specific requirements and answer questions with the iPledge Program each time the drug is dispensed. The quantity dispensed is limited, and the prescription must be picked up within a specified period of time.

Thalidomide is a drug that is used to treat multiple myeloma (a type of cancer) and erythema nodosum leprosum (a skin condition). The use of thalidomide is also restricted due to concerns about birth defects. Prescribers, patients, and pharmacies must register with the System for Thalidomide Education and Prescribing Safety (S.T.E.P.S.) program. The pharmacy must verify that the prescriber is registered with S.T.E.P.S. before dispensing the medication.

Dofetilide is used to treat irregular heart rhythms. It can cause serious complications, particularly when first starting therapy, so patients must be hospitalized to initiate therapy. Prescribers and pharmacists must register with the Tikosyn in Pharmacy System (T.I.P.S.) program, and the pharmacy must verify the prescriber's registration with the program before dispensing an outpatient prescription.

7. Verify patient using two identifiers—patient name and some other identifying information (e.g., date of birth, address, phone number). Second, patient counseling must occur with respect to state laws and patient safety. Third, patients must be given a copy of the pharmacy's patient privacy policy in compliance with HIPAA regulations. Fourth, patients' signatures are required by HIPAA when they receive the pharmacy privacy policy, by some states if they refuse patient counseling, and by some third-party payers when the patient takes possession of the prescription.

8. Pharmacy technicians may assist with Prospective Drug Utilization Review (DUR) by making sure that accurate and up-to-date information is provided for the pharmacist review (allergies, other medications, disease states or medical conditions). Depending on state regulations, pharmacy technicians should ask patients if they have any questions or would like the pharmacist to counsel them. Technicians may be very helpful in patient record maintenance.

9. Technicians might assist with disease state management and health screenings by arranging appointments and making sure the pharmacist has up-to-date information about patients. Technicians may draw up immunizations and assist with record keeping. Technicians may compound medications under the supervision of a pharmacist.

10. Pharmacists collaborate with prescribers and other health care providers to monitor patients and make adjustments or changes to medications related to a specific disease. Disease state management is most common with chronic conditions such as hypertension, hyperlipidemia, asthma, and anticoagulant therapy. Pharmacists have been able to demonstrate and document cost savings related to their services, and some payers have been willing to cover at least some of the costs of these services. A pharmacist generally completes special training to become certified to provide disease state management. Technicians may also be involved in disease state management by helping to collect and manage the data and records necessary for pharmacist monitoring.

Alphabet Soup Key

a. DUR: Drug Utilization Review

b. OBRA: Omnibus Budget Reconciliation Act

c. OTC: Over the Counter

d. PBM: Prescription Benefit Manager

e. NDC: National Drug Code

f. HMO: Health Maintenance Organization

g. HIPAA: Health Insurance Portability and Accountability Act

h. FDCA: Food, Drug, and Cosmetic Act

i. REMS: Risk Evaluation and Mitigation Strategy

j. IBS: Irritable Bowel Syndrome

k. NSAIDs: Non-Steroidal Anti-Inflammatory Drugs

l. POS: Point of Sale

m. DEA: Drug Enforcement Administration

Crosswood Puzzle Key

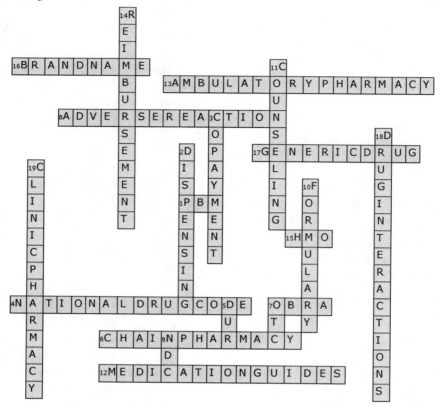

Word Search Key

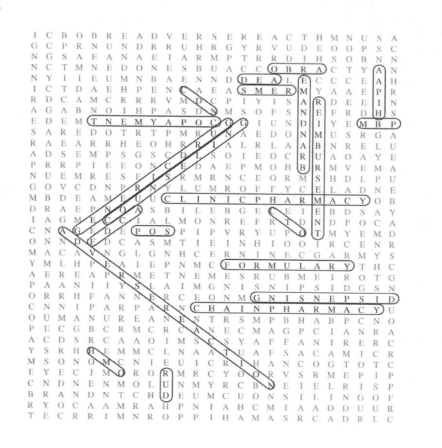

Chapter 4 Answer Keys

Multiple Choice Key

1. b. Open formulary.

2. d. All of the above.

3. d. The COO reports to the CEO.

4. d. Monitoring and evaluating patient response to medications.

5. a. They require additional resources.

6. b. Providing patient education.

7. b. Each patient is assigned to a drawer.

8. a. Recording laboratory results in the pharmacist's patient database.

Matching Key

1. D

2. A

3. E

4. F

5. B

6. I

7. J

8. G

9. H

10. C

True or False Key

1. True. Pharmacy technicians may be assigned to management or lead responsibilities.

2. False. The advantage of centralized services is that a pharmacist also has more opportunities to discuss the plan of care, answer drug information questions, and make appropriate drug therapy recommendations with other health care providers. *This is true for decentralized pharmacy services.*

3. True. The advantage of having technicians in decentralized pharmacies is that the technicians can respond quickly to any problems with medication storage cabinets.

4. False. Pharmacy technicians are not usually asked to participate on hospital committees because they do not perform tasks requiring clinical judgment. *Pharmacy technicians are often asked to participate in a variety of hospital committees based on their training and understanding of many hospital processes, especially as they relate to drug distribution systems.*

5. False. An example of an ad hoc committee is the P&T Committee. *The P&T Committee is an example of a standing committee. An example of an ad hoc committee is a committee formed to address the implementation of a new computer system for the hospital.*

6. False. Pharmacists have the responsibility to operate and maintain automated drug distribution systems because pharmacists are licensed. *This is a role well suited to trained technicians.*

7. True. Every hospital pharmacy is required by The Joint Commission to maintain a policy and procedure manual.

8. False. Studies have shown that technicians are not as accurate at checking medication carts as pharmacists. *Studies show that technicians are as accurate at checking medication carts as pharmacists.*

9. True. Technicians can screen medication orders for non-formulary status or identify if the medication is on the hospital's restricted list based on its high cost, high toxicity, or potential for over-prescribing.

10. False. Before a study is approved to be conducted in the hospital, a study protocol is developed, reviewed, and approved by the Joint Commission (TJC). *Before a study is approved to be conducted in the hospital, a study protocol is developed, reviewed, and approved by the Institutional Review Board (IRB), which often includes pharmacy representation.*

11. True. All medication storage areas in the hospital are assigned to be inspected at least monthly by pharmacy technicians.

12. False. When prescribers enter the order electronically, it is not necessary for a pharmacist to review the order for appropriateness. *Whether prescribers initiate an order verbally, enter the order electronically, or write the order, medication orders require a pharmacist to review the order for appropriateness.*

Fill in the Blank Key

1. Formulary

2. Director (or chief of pharmacy services or manager)

3. Decentralized

4. Policy and procedure

5. Medication administration record (MAR)

6. Pharmacy and Therapeutics (P&T) Committee

7. Closed

8. Pharmacy

9. The Joint Commission (TJC; formerly known as the Joint Commission on the Accreditation of Healthcare Organizations, or JCAHO)

10. Automated

11. Automated

12. Failure Mode and Effects Analysis (FMEA)

Root Cause Analysis (RCA)

Short Answer Key

1. Centralized pharmacy services handle pharmacy personnel, resources, and functions from a central location. Decentralized pharmacy services do not replace centralized pharmacy services; rather, they are used in conjunction with a central pharmacy. Decentralized pharmacy services are provided from patient care areas.

2. A closed formulary is one in which the list of available drugs is limited, and an open formulary is one in which most of the common drugs in a therapeutic class are available.

3. Formulary medications are approved based on several criteria such as indications for use, effectiveness, drug interactions, potential for errors and abuse, adverse effects, and cost.

4. If a verbal order has to be given, there are procedures for carrying out these orders to minimize errors. For example, an authorized professional within his or her scope of practice may accept a verbal order, but the order needs to be reduced to writing immediately and read back to the prescriber to clarify its accuracy. In such cases, the prescriber signs the transcription of the verbal order later to validate it.

5. In order to comply with the legal and regulatory requirements that a pharmacist must review all orders before the medication is administered, some hospitals outsource this function to remote sites.

6. The major requirements for proper labeling include patient's name, patient's location in the hospital, medication name, dose, route of administration, expiration date, and any special directions or cautionary instructions for storage or administration.

7. Medication labels are bar coded so that the nurse can scan the patient's wrist band and then the medication label to confirm that the right drug is given to the right patient.

8. An MUE is commonly performed with medications that fall into one or more categories identified by the hospital, including high-use drugs, high-cost drugs, and high-risk drugs. Data is collected to evaluate the appropriate use of these drugs, including appropriate indications, dose, route, and clinical response. After the MUE data is collected on a predefined number of patients, the results are tabulated and presented to the appropriate health care providers and committees. Depending on the results, appropriate recommendations and actions are taken. For example, if the data shows many patients are receiving doses too high based on the indication and renal function, recommendations and actions may be provided that include education and training to health care providers on the appropriate dosing criteria for this medication. Another action may be to give the pharmacist authority to automatically change the dose based on approved criteria by the P&T Committee. No matter what technique or data source is used to evaluate the process, the primary goal is to identify areas for improvement and implement strategies or needed changes in the process to improve the medication management system.

9. The benefits of accreditation include strengthening community confidence in the quality and safety of care, treatment, and services; provision of a competitive edge in the marketplace; improvement of risk management and risk reduction; provision of education on good practices to improve business operations; provision of professional advice and counsel; enhancement of staff education; staff recruitment and development; and recognition by select insurers and other third parties.

10. Quality improvement (QI) is a formal or systematic approach to analyzing the performance of a system or process. Quality control (QC) is a process of checks and balances (or procedures) that are followed during the manufacturing of a product or provision of a service to ensure that the end products or services meet or exceed specified standards (e.g., zero errors, zero problems).

Alphabet Soup Key

a. QC: Quality Control

b. QI: Quality Improvement

c. CQI: Continuous Quality Improvement

d. TQM: Total Quality Management

e. FMEA: Failure Mode and Effects Analysis

f. RCA: Root Cause Analysis

g. ISMP: The Institute for Safe Medication Practices

h. ASHP: American Society of Health-System Pharmacists

i. IHI: Institute for Healthcare Improvement

j. TJC: The Joint Commission

k. IOM: Institute of Medicine

l. AHRQ: Agency for Healthcare Research and Quality

m. CMS: Centers for Medicare and Medicaid Services

n. NCQA: National Committee for Quality Assurance

o. HMO: Health Maintenance Organization

p. P&T Committee: Pharmacy and Therapeutics Committee

q. MAR: Medication Administration Record

r. MUE: Medication Use Evaluation

s. IV: Intravenous

t. CEO: Chief Executive Officer

u. COO: Chief Operating Officer

v. CPOE: Computerized Physician (or Prescriber) Order Entry

w. IRB: Institutional Review Board

Word Search Key

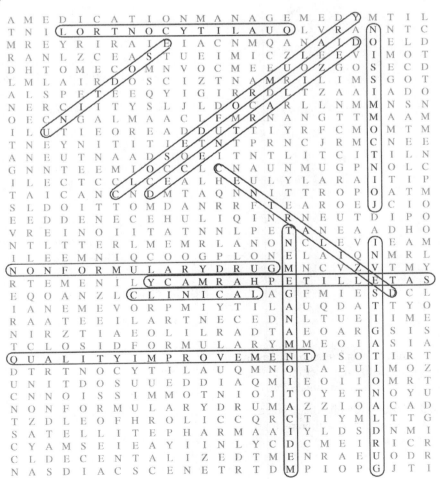

Chapter 5 Answer Keys

Multiple Choice Key

1. d. All of the above.

2. d. All of the above.

3. d. Nurse.

4. d. All of the above.

5. b. The organism(s) identified in the cultures.

6. d. All of the above.

7. e. None of the above.

8. a. Oral acetaminophen and diphenhydramine.

9. b. Filgrastim.

10. d. All of the above.

Matching I Key

1. C

2. D

3. B

4. E

5. A

Matching II Key

1. D

2. G

3. A

4. C

5. E

6. F

7. B

True or False Key

1. False. Patients first began receiving infusion therapy in the home, rather than in an institutional setting, in the late 1950s. *This practice started in the late 1970s.*

2. False. The major goal of home care pharmacy practice is to provide safe and effective infusion therapy in the home *that is also cost effective.*

3. False. An intake coordinator for home health care is usually a *nurse, but a pharmacy technician could be trained for this responsibility.*

4. False. It should only take a quick visit for the nurse to train the patient or caregiver about how to administer medications. *Several nursing visits are often required to ensure that the patient can perform medication administration and other procedures properly.*

5. True. Anti-infectives account for the majority of pharmaceuticals used in home infusion therapy.

6. False. Red Man Syndrome is a reaction from rapid infusion of *vancomycin* that causes a redness or flushing of the head and torso. *Vancomycin should be infused at a rate of no greater than 1 gram over 60 minutes to prevent Red Man Syndrome.*

7. True. Normal saline, commonly used to flush the catheter before and after the infusion of medication, is incompatible with amphotericin B. Mixing the two results in a precipitate.

8. True. To avoid making parenteral nutrition bags that cannot be used, the technician should coordinate mixing of a patient's parenteral nutrition to follow scheduled laboratory blood draws and pharmacist and nursing assessments and visits.

9. False. Enteral nutrition is the administration of specialized formulas that are high in required nutrients *through the stomach or part of the small intestine (jejunum) to meet a patient's nutritional needs.*

10. False. Ninety percent of home care narcotic orders are for *morphine.*

11. True. Most products prepared for use by home care patients fall into risk level 2 (medium risk) because they are stored for more than 7 days.

12. False. For drugs to be given via an ambulatory infusion device, at least *24-hour* stability at room temperature or warmer is required.

Fill in the Blank Key

1. Extravasation

2. Universal precautions

3. Smart

4. Elastomeric balloon system

5. Patient controlled analgesia (PCA)

6. Cephalosporin

7. Red Man Syndrome

8. A precipitate

9. Total parenteral nutrition (TPN)

10. 797

11. 2

12. Biological safety cabinet (BSC)

Short Answer Key

1. It is cost effective for some patients to receive infusions at home rather than to be hospitalized for infusions. It can be a hardship for patients' families too. Home infusion therapy is safe, effective, and less expensive; it also allows patients to resume normal lifestyles and work activities while recovering from illness. Treating patients at home has the advantage, in some cases, of helping them to avoid the risk of hospital-acquired infections such as hospital-acquired pneumonia.

2. The care plan includes methods of assessment of therapy and complications of therapy. Frequency of visits for assessment of patient status and home care supplies is determined by stability of patient, stability of patient medications, and frequency of lab work needed for patient care in order to accomplish the goal of a successful course of therapy without any adverse events. Once home care therapy is completed, the patient is discharged from the home care service.

3. A *case manager* will mediate the location of the therapy. Once the decision has been made to send a patient home, a *social worker or a discharge planner* contacts the home care agency and initiates the process. The discharge planner is often a registered nurse with home care experience, and he or she will begin preparing the patient for home therapy.

   An *intake coordinator* at the home care company receives the patient referral. This person is responsible for retrieving the patient's contact information (address, phone number, etc.), diagnosis, requested home care therapy, pertinent medical data, and insurance information. The intake coordinator is often a nurse but may also be a technician specially trained for the job.

   A *registered nurse* trained in home infusion makes the initial patient visit and teaches the patient about the administration of medication. Secondary members are involved for specialized services and *include registered dietitians, respiratory therapists, social workers, physical and occupational therapists, and certified nursing assistants (CNA).*

The *physician* is the leader of the team, and he or she is ultimately responsible for the care of the patient. The *infusion nurse* and *pharmacist* work together to coordinate patient supplies, develop a plan of care, monitor and document the patient's status, communicate with the physician, coordinate physician orders, and make appropriate interventions.

The *pharmacy technician* prepares medications for home infusion, generating medication labels, compounding, preparing, and labeling medications; and maintaining the compounding room and drug storage areas. Pharmacy technicians are often responsible for managing the warehouse and inventory of non-drug supplies, keeping track of accounts receivable, picking and packaging supplies for shipment to patients, and arranging for delivery of supplies to patients.

The pharmacist is also an educator, responsible for instructing the patient and the nurse on the drugs being administered. Important additional clinical pharmacy roles are pharmacokinetic dosing of vancomycin and aminoglycosides, providing nutritional support services, and having input in the selection of the most appropriate drug for the patient. The pharmacist is the drug information source for all other team members.

Although not active in direct patient care, the *reimbursement specialist* is key to the economic viability of the company. The reimbursement department is the interface among the insurer, the home infusion company, and the patient. Many companies employ a *patient service representative* who is responsible for controlling the patient's inventory of supplies and screening for problems. Not to be forgotten as team members are the *patient and the caregivers.* In home care, much of the burden falls on their shoulders. They must be involved in the decision making and the development of the care plan. The patient's right to be involved is clearly stated in the rights and responsibilities document that is presented on the initial visit.

4. Parenteral nutrition is *intravenous* nutrition that provides a patient with all of the fluid and essential nutrients he or she needs when oral hydration is difficult or impossible. Enteral nutrition is the administration of specialized formulas that are high in required nutrients *through the stomach or part of the small intestine (jejunum)* to meet a patient's nutritional needs.

5. Five types of infusion systems are available for patients to use at home: (1) minibag infusion via gravity system, (2) syringe infusion via syringe device, (3) syringe infusion via IV push method, (4) rate-restricted IV administration set systems, and (5) ambulatory electronic infusion pumps. There are a great number of considerations

in choosing the correct infusion type for a particular patient. They include product design, reliability, compatibility and stability, ease of staff training, nursing interaction time, pharmacy filling time, ability of device to minimize complications, ability of device to mini-mize waste, storage space needed at provider's facility, storage space needed in patient's home, manufacturer and/or distributor support, ease of product disposal, inventory costs, product efficacy, availability, downtime and repair cost, and ease of patient/caregiver training.

Crosswood Puzzle Key

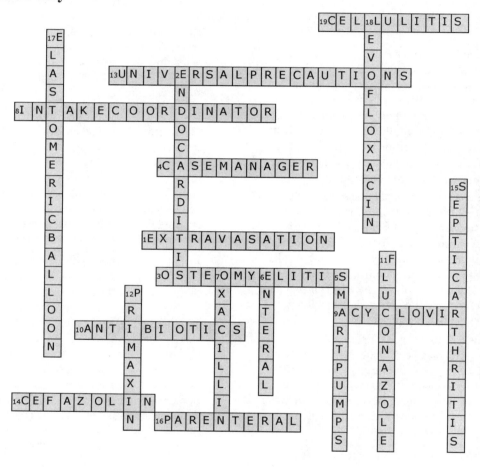

Word Search Key

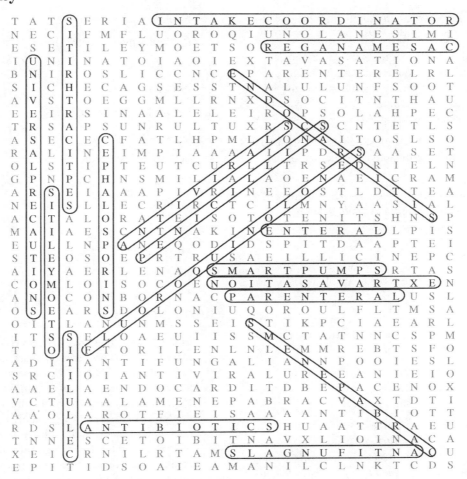

Chapter 6 Answer Keys

Multiple Choice Key

1. c. Both a and b.

2. c. Radioactivity.

3. e. All of the above.

4. a. A 2- or 3-hour travel distance.

5. The answers in a and c and d are true.

6. b. The amount of radioactivity that will be administered to the patient.

7. d. Pharmacist.

8. c. A segregated area away from traffic to comply with sterile product compounding guidelines.

9. b. Radiopharmaceutical kit.

10. a. BPS.

Matching Key

1. H

2. G

3. D

4. F

5. E

6. C

7. A

8. B

True or False Key

1. True. The human body contains small amounts of radioactive carbon and potassium.

2. True. The functional information provided by nuclear medicine studies is used to augment the anatomic information that is obtained by traditional imaging modalities such as x-ray, computed tomography (CT), or magnetic resonance imaging (MRI).

3. False. Radiopharmaceuticals must be compounded on a *daily* basis due to the radioactive component of the products.

4. False. The *nonrestricted* areas are the general areas of the pharmacy where the staff and visitors can be assured of having limited to no contact with radioactive materials.

5. True. Very often, pharmacy technicians are responsible for maintaining appropriate recordkeeping and radioactive waste disposal.

6. False. When dispensing radiopharmaceuticals, the activity for the dose must be accurate at the time the material is *to be injected into the patient.*

7. True. After every product prepared is compounded, it undergoes quality control testing before any patient dose is released from the pharmacy.

8. False. Common quality control tests performed in a nuclear pharmacy *are quick (generally less than 1 minute to complete) and easy to perform. Generally, quality control testing is a task assigned to a pharmacy technician or a very advanced member of the delivery staff.*

9. True. The sources of regulatory compliance involve the Nuclear Regulatory Commission (NRC) and the Department of Transportation (DOT).

10. False. Currently, *pharmacists* are responsible for all aspects of the preparation and dispensing of radiopharmaceuticals used for therapeutic purposes *due to the risk involved for both the pharmacist and the patient if errors are made in these doses.*

11. False. The FDA *"Green Book"* is a listing of all animal drug products that have been approved for safety and effectiveness.

12. True. A fairly innocuous drug used in the canine population (aspirin, for example) can be lethal to cats because they have a deficiency in the normal metabolic pathway for this drug.

Fill in the Blank Key

1. Nuclear pharmacy

2. Radiopharmaceuticals

3. Radon

4. Activity units (mCi)

5. Geiger Mueller (GM)

6. Dose calibrator

7. Scintillation detector

8. Ligand

9. Tc-99m

10. Unit dose

11. Shielding

12. "Green Book"

Short Answer Key

1. In the 1940s, Dr. John Christian recognized the potential relationship between pharmacy and the use of radioactivity. He established a series of training courses at Purdue University that are still in existence today. Captain Briner established the first radiopharmacy at the NIH in 1958, and he is widely recognized in the nuclear pharmacy community as the "Father of Radiopharmacy." In the 1970s, several schools of pharmacy created formalized educational programs, recognizing that pharmacists with specialty training would be best prepared to provide the services needed to support the nuclear medicine community. In 1978, nuclear pharmacy was recognized by the American Pharmaceutical Association (APhA) as the first specialty area of pharmacy practice, with development of a board certification specialty examination (BCNP). Currently, more than 500 nuclear pharmacists have earned board certification. There are three major chain nuclear pharmacies with more than 200 locations and more than 100 independently owned nuclear pharmacies throughout the United States today.

2. Radioactivity involves the transfer of excess energy into a radioactive emission. Within an atom, the nucleus contains protons (positive [+] charge) and neutrons (neutral charge). Surrounding the nucleus are electrons (negative [-] charge). Some atoms contain an imbalance in the ratios between the protons and neutrons within the nucleus, which makes them unstable. In order to return to a more stable state, the atom must release some of the excess energy. In some atoms, this excess energy

is given off as a radioactive emission. Radioactive material has a distinct characteristic called a half-life. The half-life of a radioactive material is the amount of time that it takes for one-half of the material to give up its excess energy in the form of a radioactive emission.

Most medical applications use radioactive materials that are created in a nuclear reactor or an accelerator. Medical isotopes are produced using the same technology, but on a significantly smaller scale. In a reactor, a large atom (usually uranium) is split in a process called fission. Some of the byproducts generated are radioactive and can be collected and purified to be used in medical applications. In an accelerator, a stable atom is bombarded with a positively or negatively charged particle that creates an imbalance in the atom. These agents have shorter half-lives and are more useful for performing nuclear medicine imaging.

3. Nuclear medicine plays an important role in the diagnosis and treatment of disease. Diagnostic nuclear medicine studies involve attaching a small amount of radioactive material to a compound (called a ligand) that is known to behave a certain way when it is introduced into the body. Once administered, the ligand moves through the patient's body, following a physiologic process that occurs within that patient (e.g., elimination of waste through the kidney, remodeling of bone structure, and blood flow to the heart muscle). As the ligand moves through the body, the radioactive material gives off a radioactive emission called a gamma photon, which passes out of the patient's body and into a detector located near the patient. The radioactive emissions are detected and mapped to identify how the tracer moves through the patient's body. From this data, physicians can gain information about how the particular organ is working as well as the physiologic process that should be occurring.

As an example, in renal imaging, the organ of interest would be the kidney, while the physiologic process of concern would be excretion of waste products. The agents used for renal imaging are taken up by the kidney just like typical waste products in the blood. The agent is removed from the kidney in the urine and moves to the bladder. By watching the movement of the radioactive emissions as the agent moves through the kidney, one could determine if there is adequate blood flow to the kidneys, if the kidneys are functioning properly, and if urine is able to pass out of the kidney and into the bladder. The functional information provided by nuclear medicine studies is used to augment the anatomic information that is obtained by traditional imaging modalities such as x-ray, computed tomography (CT), or magnetic resonance imaging (MRI).

Nuclear medicine is also used as a form of treatment for certain diseases by taking advantage of the destructive effects of certain types of radioactive emissions to provide localized treatment of disease. The most common example is the use of a radioactive form of iodide for the treatment of thyroid diseases such as overactive thyroid or thyroid cancer. The thyroid gland typically takes iodide from the bloodstream to make thyroid hormones that play an important role in maintaining basic functions of the body. When administering a radioactive form of the iodide molecule, the thyroid gland takes up the radioactive iodide molecule just like it takes up the normal iodine molecule. Once in the gland, the radioactive emissions from the molecule cause damage to the thyroid tissue. In patients with an overactive thyroid, this is enough to return function back to normal levels. The dose is substantially higher in thyroid cancer. The goal is to completely damage all thyroid tissue, which treats the cancer and prevents disease recurrence.

There are more than 100 different nuclear medicine imaging procedures available today, with approximately 16 million imaging and therapy procedures performed annually in the United States alone; the majority are related to cardiac and oncology applications. These procedures can be performed on any patient population, including pediatric patients.

4. Depending on state regulations, telephone orders can be taken by pharmacists and, in some cases, pharmacy technicians. Pharmacists are primarily responsible for the compounding of radiopharmaceuticals in most nuclear pharmacies. Pharmacy technicians are primarily responsible for taking the batch of prepared radiopharmaceutical (prepared in the compounding area) and withdrawing a designated amount of the material from the source vial into one or more patient doses. One common procedure performed in most nuclear pharmacies is the isolation and radiolabeling of white blood cells that have been withdrawn from a patient in the hospital nuclear medicine department to assist in the detection of the body's infection sites. In many pharmacies, both pharmacists and pharmacy technicians are responsible for the isolation and radiolabeling process.

Because all doses dispensed must be delivered to the end user at a facility outside of the radiopharmacy, a large area of the pharmacy is dedicated to the safe packaging and transport of these doses. Driver/courier staff members in the pharmacy are responsible for ensuring that the dose containers are not contaminated with external radioactive material, placing the correct doses in appropriate shipping containers, completing inventory before shipping, and following the appropriate regulatory requirements for shipping radioactive materials.

Technicians are sometimes involved in these activities once they have completed the dose drawing process to expedite the packaging and transport process. Once the radioactive waste (which is also biohazardous because it was most likely injected into a patient's bloodstream and may have some blood contamination) has reached appropriate levels of radioactivity, it is sent to a medical waste facility for disposal. This is a highly regulated area of the pharmacy; very often, pharmacy technicians are responsible for maintaining appropriate recordkeeping and waste disposal.

5. As in any other pharmacy that provides compounding services, the role of the technician varies. Technicians are responsible for the actual compounding activities in some situations. For technicians who would like to work in this environment, the most difficult issue is finding a location that specializes in providing pharmacy services for an animal population.

Internet Research Key

1. This web page is updated frequently (within a few days).

2. a. Spotlight information—latest information on hot topics such as:

    i. Food Registry for Industry Pet Food.
    ii. CVM Updates.
    iii. Salmonella and Turtle Safety.
    iv. Bovine Spongiform Encephalopathy.

  b. Recalls & Alerts

  c. Approvals & Clearances for new drugs

  d. CVM Information (Center for Veterinary Medicine)

  e. Development & Approval Process

  f. Guidance, Compliance & Enforcement

  g. News & Events

  h. Products

  i. Resources for You

  j. Safety & Health

  k. Science & Research

  l. Research Areas, Publications

It would be helpful for compounding pharmacies to know the latest news, and to be able to look up drug approvals. There is also a "Contact Us" area for specific questions.

3. EXAMPLE

a. Nuclear Education Online (NEO): This educational consortium is between the University of Arkansas for Medical Sciences and the University of New Mexico College of Pharmacy.

b. This self-study program represents a minimum of 10 weeks of supervised, experiential training with an Authorized Nuclear Pharmacist preceptor. Candidates with nuclear pharmacy experience should complete the program in not less than 20 weeks. No specific schedule or curriculum is required for program completion.

c. Program Costs: Tuition for the NPT training program is $1800, which includes online instruction, aseptic technique DVD and manual, and competency assessments. Students who are unable to complete the education program may request a full or partial refund.

d. ACPE Accreditation: This program provides pharmacy participants 35 contact hours. These continuing education (CE) credits are provided for participants enrolled as of April 26, 2006. To receive credit, the student must complete all program evaluation forms and pass the course final with a grade of 70% or better. Statements of credit will be issued by the University of Arkansas for Medical Sciences (UAMS), College of Pharmacy (COP) CE office within 10 business days of receipt of necessary materials from NEO.

Chapter 7 Answer Keys

Multiple Choice Key

1. b. Secondary references.

2. d. All of the above. Cost questions are particularly complex because there are so many factors to consider beyond the simple cost of the medication.

3. d. Ask the patient to wait a moment while you check on something, and then quietly check with the pharmacist before the patient makes the purchase and leaves the pharmacy. *You and the pharmacist should work as a team for patient safety. Any potential problems should be reported to the pharmacist as soon as possible.*

4. b. First consult tertiary references, then secondary references, and finally primary references.

5. c. Tertiary references.

6. d. A three-volume set that provides medication informa-

tion for health care professionals and patients.

7. d. All of the above.

8. e. None of the above.

9. d. USP Pharmacist's Pharmacopeia.

10. c. The Natural Medicines Comprehensive Database.

Matching Key

NOTE: All of these questions can be answered by a pharmacist. Knowledgeable pharmacy technicians can answer many questions, but whenever the technician is not sure of the answer, the question should be referred to the pharmacist. Sometimes questions may be answered partially by a technician, with follow-up from a pharmacist. Keep in mind that some questions are actually just a reason to start a dialogue with a pharmacist, with the "real" question following introductory conversation after the patient feels comfortable with the pharmacist. Screening questions for the pharmacist can be challenging. Individual pharmacists may feel differently about the answers given below. It is very important for the technician and the pharmacist to communicate well together and have an understanding about what questions the pharmacist is comfortable having the technician answer.

1. B. What is the brand name of warfarin? Factual answer—can be looked up.

2. A. Do Naprosyn and Aleve contain the same active ingredient? Seems like a factual answer upon first glance, but answer might involve different salt forms of naproxen with regard to onset and absorption, so pharmacist should answer.

3. B. Who manufactures Enbrel? Factual answer—can be looked up.

4. B. Is Prilosec available as a generic? Is it a prescription or over-the-counter (OTC) product? Factual answer— can be looked up.

5. B. What dosage forms of Imitrex are available in your pharmacy? Factual answer—can be looked up and tech should be able to look at wholesaler information to see if other forms are available for order.

6. A. Is Zoloft available as a liquid? If so, what size and concentration are available? Seems factual answer—can be looked up. However, special doses can be compounded and a pharmacist would be the best resource for that information.

7. B. What are the prices of Adalat CC and Procardia XL? Factual answer—can be looked up.

8. B_C. How long is the shortage of albumin expected to last? This answer is really site-specific. In some hospital

pharmacies, pharmacy technicians are utilized as buyers and are the best resource for this information. Many hospitals still utilize pharmacists in the buyer role; in that case, the pharmacist would be the best resource.

9. B. Should Lovenox be stored in the refrigerator? Factual answer—can be looked up.

10. B. How long is a flu shot stable after it is drawn up in a syringe? Factual answer—can be looked up.

11. B. How many milliliters are in an ounce? Factual answer—can be looked up.

12. B. How should ampicillin be reconstituted? Factual answer—can be looked up.

13. B. In what controlled substance schedule is zolpidem (Ambien)? Factual answer—can be looked up.

14. A. Can Tiazac be substituted for Cardizem CD (is it AB rated)? This question can be looked up, but there may be some therapeutic discussion on the differences of the two medication brands and benefits versus differences of the various medications in this class.

15. B. How many times can a prescription be transferred from one store to another? Factual answer—can be looked up.

16. B. Where can I find the phone number for Sanofi Aventis? Factual answer—can be looked up.

17. B. When will the patent for Lipitor expire? Factual answer—can be looked up.

18. B. Where can I get more Lovenox teaching kits? Factual answer—can be looked up.

19. B. Where can I find the Vaccine Information Sheet for the influenza vaccine? Factual answer—can be looked up.

True or False Key

1. False. If you are asked a question about the usual dose of a medication, you may answer the question if you know the answer. *In general, if a question requires specific knowledge about a medication and/or professional judgment, it should be answered by a pharmacist. In this case, how do you know which usual dose is being requested? What seems like an easy question can quickly become more involved. In this case, the dose requested might be for one of many indications for a particular medication with many different "usual doses," depending upon the indication, or this might be for a child, an adult, a person with compromised kidney function, or a pregnant person.*

2. True. Consumers may not understand which questions a pharmacy technician can answer and which should be referred to the pharmacist. *Often consumers are unaware of the differences in educational preparation between pharmacy technicians and pharmacists. You should always check with the pharmacist about any question that is not clearly a technician question, or a technician question that you cannot answer with 100% confidence that you are correct.*

3. False. The term "scope of practice" means any work you have been allowed to do in your work environment. *"Scope of practice" refers to what you may legally do in your position. It is important to know your scope of practice as a pharmacy technician in your state.*

4. False. All drug information requests should be answered in written and referenced format. *Depending on the question, the requestor, and the depth of information needed, the format of the answer may vary from a short verbal response to a detailed and written response, including references or any combination of responses such as an immediate verbal response followed by a more detailed response.*

5. False. When answering questions from patients, you will be more respected as an expert if you use medical terminology as much as possible. *Medical terminology should be avoided, and the response should be put it into language that patients can understand.*

6. False. If you have heard a pharmacist answer a clinical question many times, it is okay for you to give the answer you know that the pharmacist would have given. *Clinical questions must be answered by a pharmacist. There may be many times that the answer is the same, but keep in mind there may be circumstances where the answer is not the same.*

7. True. Answers to many medication questions may be found in a multitude of references. *Depending on the pharmacist and the work site, many different references would suffice for the same question. Pharmacists tend to have a "go to" reference. Some pharmacists use PDAs such as iPODS to store many reference books for quick referrals.*

8. True. Many references are available in several formats, such as "hard copy," online, or downloaded to computers or hand held devices. *Facts and Comparisons, Lexi-Comp, Orange Book, Natural Medicines Comprehensive Database, and many more offer several formats.*

9. False. If a physician's name is associated with Internet information, it is probably a reliable Internet site. *Internet sites should be certified or associated with real government oversight such as the FDA. Physicians and other health care professionals have been associated with unethical health claims on the Internet in order to sell products or information to consumers.*

10. True. One of the most important steps in answering a drug information question is follow-up such as inquiries to the requestor about whether the information was useful and/or if it was answered. This will ensure that the response was complete.

11. True. The Red Book is a good source for lists of sugar, lactose, galactose, alcohol-free products, sulfite-containing products, and medications that shouldn't be crushed.

Fill in the Blank Key

1. PubMed
2. MedlinePlus
3. Tertiary
4. Package insert
5. Lexi-Comp
6. Red Book
7. Orange Book
8. CDC
9. Poison Control Center
10. FDA

Short Answer Key

1. Find out information about the requestor such as his or her name and background (lay person, physician, pharmacist, nurse, etc.) so that the response is tailored to the knowledge base of the requestor. Find out about the purpose of the request so that it may be determined if the response requires judgment, necessitating the expertise of a pharmacist. It is important to know if the request is for general information or if it pertains to a specific patient. If the question involves a specific patient, the pharmacist will need to obtain background information in order to respond to the question. The urgency of the request and the extent of the information needed should also be determined so that an appropriate amount of time is allotted to answer the request.

2. Classifying the type of request helps to narrow the search and makes the search process more efficient. It is critical that technicians differentiate questions that fall within their scope of practice from those that may be answered only by a pharmacist. There are several clas-

sifications listed below, although some questions may fall in other categories not listed.

Identification and availability—Although it is appropriate for a technician to obtain technical information about availability (e.g., anticipated length/reasons for a shortage), questions that require clinical knowledge such as therapeutic alternatives must be answered by a pharmacist.

Allergies—For allergy questions, the pharmacist must obtain more patient-specific information such as a description of the allergy and the condition being treated. Clinical judgment is required.

Dosing and administration—Answers to dosing and administration questions depend on many factors. If the question relates to the indication for use and patient-specific information (e.g., age, weight, and kidney and liver function), clinical judgment is necessary.

Compatibility—Often more information is needed (e.g., doses, concentrations, fluids, and type of IV lines). For some compatibility questions, a pharmacist must interpret information found in a reference and apply it to the situation.

Drug interactions—Drug interaction questions are complex and require patient-specific information and interpretation by a pharmacist in order to apply the significance of a potential interaction to a specific patient.

Side effects—Package inserts and textbooks provide lists of side effects that are often difficult to interpret and convey. Also, a pharmacist must interpret whether the request is being made because an adverse event is suspected with one or more medications.

Pregnancy and lactation—Pregnancy and lactation questions are complicated because more information is needed about the patient, the stage of pregnancy, and/or age of the infant. A pharmacist must interpret the findings and apply them to the specific situation.

Therapeutic use—The use of drugs for non-FDA approved uses often requires evaluation and interpretation of the literature and clinical judgment.

3. Primary references are original research articles published in scientific journals such as the *American Journal of Health-System Pharmacy (AJHP)* or the *Journal of the American Pharmacists Association (JAPhA)*. An advantage of primary references is that the information is directly from the researchers and is usually very detailed. The disadvantage of primary references is that the information may be more detailed than necessary for the request, and it may take time to find answers to specific questions.

Secondary references include indexing systems such as Medline, which provide a list of journal articles on the topic that is being searched. The advantage of secondary references is that the information is usually very current. A disadvantage is that the listed journal articles are not always readily available to a pharmacy.

Tertiary references present documented information in a condensed and compact format. They may include textbooks, compendia (e.g., American Hospital Formulary Service Drug Information [AHFS DI] and Drug Facts & Comparisons), computerized systems such as Micromedex® Clinical Information System, review articles, or information found on the Internet. Tertiary references are the most commonly used references because they are easy to use, convenient, readily accessible, concise, and compact. Disadvantages of tertiary references are that information may not be current, the information may contain errors, and the level of detail on a specific topic may not be deep enough due to space restrictions.

4. Material Safety Data Sheets (MSDS) are information sheets provided by manufacturers for chemicals or drugs that may be hazardous in the workplace. The primary purpose of the MSDS is to provide information about the specific hazards of the chemicals or drugs used at the worksite, to provide guidelines for their safe use, and to provide recommendations to treat an exposure or clean up a spill. Materials commonly encountered in pharmacies that require MSDS information at the workplace site include chemotherapy agents (e.g., doxorubicin and methotrexate), hormonal agents (e.g., diethylstilbestrol), volatile or explosive agents (e.g., isopropyl alcohol and ethyl alcohol), and chemicals stocked for compounding purposes (even innocuous things like olive oil and simple syrup). Material Safety Data Sheets contain information that may be used to answer the following questions: What precautions must be taken when preparing and dispensing doxorubicin? Where should isopropyl alcohol be stored? How should an employee exposed to doxorubicin be immediately treated? How should a chemotherapy spill be cleaned?

5. Government sites such as the FDA are reputable. Pharmaceutical manufacturers, which represent FDA-approved medications, are reliable since they have only FDA-approved content on them. *Check at the bottom of the web page to see if and when the site has been reviewed and by whom.* Most pharmacy and medical organizations have their information reviewed by experts in the particular field and are therefore considered reputable, but sites can contain erroneous and/or misleading information, especially if a product is being sold. Most of the publishers of the references that have been identified in this chapter have developed Internet versions

Part 1

of their resources. Internet versions are advantageous because the end user no longer has to update hard copy references, and they can be accessed with a username and password from any computer with Internet access.

6. In a very busy pharmacy, it is important to make sure everyone receives proper information in the most efficient but complete method possible. Make some notes, including the patient name, the contact information, and the actual question; ask if the customer would prefer that the pharmacist call her or if she would like to wait in line. Since the information she requests requires a pharmacist's judgment, you should make sure she will get answers as soon as possible.

7. The PDR is not comprehensive and only contains information on select brand name drugs. The information is written by the manufacturer and approved by the FDA. It only contains information about FDA-approved uses of the drug. It does not provide comparative information of that drug with similar medications. Therefore, the PDR may not be as useful as other resources in comparing products. Information about generic medications is typically not included.

Alphabet Soup Key

a. CDC: Centers for Disease Control

b. NIH: National Institutes for Health

c. CDER: Center for Drug Evaluation and Research

d. FDA: Food and Drug Administration

e. AHFS DI: American Hospital Formulary Service Drug Information

f. AJHP: American Journal of Health-System Pharmacy

g. JAPhA: Journal of the American Pharmacists Association

h. ASHP: American Society of Health-System Pharmacists

i. OTC: Over-the-Counter

j. PDR: Physicians' Desk Reference

k. APhA: American Pharmacists Association

l. MSDS: Material Safety Data Sheets

m. AAPCC: American Association of Poison Control Centers

n. NLM: National Library of Medicine

o. ISMP: Institute for Safe Medication Practices

Internet Research Key

1. The best web site for checking on necessary preparations for travel to Peru is noted here: http://wwwnc.cdc.gov/travel/destinations/peru.aspx

   Travel recommendations may change from time to time. The recommendations for travel to Peru in 2010 are as follows:

Routine vaccines, as they are often called, such as for influenza, chickenpox (or varicella), polio, measles/mumps/rubella (MMR), and diphtheria/pertussis/tetanus (DPT) are given at all stages of life; see the childhood and adolescent immunization schedule and routine adult immunization schedule.

Routine vaccines are recommended even if you do not travel. Although childhood diseases, such as measles, rarely occur in the United States, they are still common in many parts of the world. A traveler who is not vaccinated would be at risk for infection.

Malaria

Areas of Peru with Malaria: All departments <2000 m (6,561 ft) except none in Arequipa, Moquegua, Puno, and Tacna. Present in Puerto Maldonado. No malaria in highland tourist areas (Cuzco, Machu Picchu, and Lake Titicaca).. (more information)

If you will be visiting an area of Peru with malaria, you will need to discuss with your doctor the best ways for you to avoid getting sick with malaria. Ways to prevent malaria include the following:

- Taking a prescription antimalarial drug

- Using insect repellent and wearing long pants and sleeves to prevent mosquito bites

- Sleeping in air-conditioned or well-screened rooms or using bednets

If you are traveling to Lima or the coastal areas south of Lima, the risk of malaria is low and taking an antimalarial drug is not recommended. However, you should protect yourself from mosquito bites (see below).

If you are traveling to an area of malaria in any other part of Peru, all of the following antimalarial drugs are equal options for preventing malaria: Atovaquone/proguanil, doxycycline, or mefloquine.

Note: Chloroquine is NOT an effective antimalarial drug in Peru and should not be taken to prevent malaria in this region.

To find out more information on malaria throughout the world, you can use the interactive CDC malaria map. You can search or browse countries, cities, and place names for more specific malaria risk information and the recommended prevention medicines for that area.

2. Details for starting an accredited technician training program are found at these web sites:

http://www.ashp.org/Import/ACCREDITATION/TechnicianAccreditation/StartingaTrainingProgram.aspx

http://www.ashp.org/Import/ACCREDITATION/TechnicianAccreditation/ApplyAccreditation.aspx

The form for applying for ASHP accreditation is located at:

http://www.ashp.org/Import/ACCREDITATION/TechnicianAccreditation/ApplyAccreditation.aspx

3. At the time of the writing of this workbook, these drugs were on the shortages list:

Acetaminophen Suppositories	September 01, 2010
Acetaminophen/dichloralphenazone/ isometheptene	September 03, 2010
Acetazolamide Injection	August 17, 2010
Acyclovir Injection	August 30, 2010
Acyclovir Capsules and Tablets	July 08, 2010

By clicking on each name of the drug, details regarding the shortages may be found.

An example of the type of information you will find is below:

• Actavis has Feverall 80 mg suppositories (NDC 00472-1200-06) and 120 mg (NDC 00472-1201-06) in 6 count packages available. Feverall 120 mg in 50 count packages (NDC 00472-1201-50) are available in limited quantities.All other Feverall suppository presentations are on intermittent back order and the company is releasing product as it becomes available.

• G&W Laboratories has acetaminophen 120 mg suppositories on back order with an estimated release date of early-September, 2010. All 325 mg and 650 mg presentations are on an intermittent back order and the company is releasing product as it becomes available. The 650 mg presentation in 500 count has been discontinued.

• Perrigo has all acetaminophen suppository presentations on back order with an estimated release date of late-September, 2010. The 120 mg presentation in 50 count has been discontinued.

• Watson has all acetaminophen suppository presentations on back order with an estimated release date of mid-September, 2010.

4. ISMP will update suggestions for error prevention. Four examples (and there are many more) are:

i. Use Standard Order Sets and use guidelines in developing these sets:

"If standard order sets are not carefully designed, reviewed, and maintained to reflect best practices and ensure clear communication, they may actually contribute to errors. The ISMP Guidelines for Standard Order Sets has been developed to help organizations ensure that the elements of safe order communication have been followed when designing paper-based or electronic order sets. The guidelines focus primarily on medication orders within order sets but also cover general aspects related to the design, approval, and maintenance of all standard order sets. ISMP recommends using this checklist to guide the design and evaluation of standard order sets before granting approval for use."

ii. Use the Risk assessment tool for ambulatory pharmacy:
"Welcome to the Risk Assessment for Medication Safety
With the release of Improving Medication Safety in Community Pharmacy: Assessing Risk and Opportunities for Change, community pharmacies now have access to a coordinated, extensive set of tools designed to reduce medication errors. The Risk document is designed to help community pharmacies take a process-driven, system-based approach to address this critical issue.

The tools were developed by the Institute for Safe Medication Practices (ISMP) with grant support from National Association of Chain Drug Stores Foundation and the AstraZeneca Medical Group."

iii. Implement the recommendations in this paper:
"PROCEEDINGS FROM THE ISMP SUMMIT ON THE USE OF SMART INFUSION PUMPS: GUIDELINES FOR SAFE IMPLEMENTATION AND USE"

iv. Follow the guidelines for safe labeling of medications found in this article:
"Principles of Designing a Medication Label for Community and Mail Order Pharmacy Prescription Packages Document"

Chapter 8 Answer Keys

Multiple Choice Key

1. b. "An individual working in a pharmacy who, under the supervision of a licensed pharmacist, assists in pharmacy activities that do not require the professional judgment of a pharmacist."

2. d. All of the above.

3. d. All of the above.

4. a. Ensure that the recipient party hears the same message, both in content and intent, as the deliverer and that the intended result of that message is achieved.

5. d. All of the above.

6. d. Must manage personal feelings while recognizing and considering the feelings of their patients.

7. a. Transmitting, receiving, and processing information.

8. e. None of the above.

9. e. None of the above.

10. d. All of the above.

Matching Key

1. D
2. B
3. C
4. A
5. D
6. C
7. B
8. A

True or False Key

1. True. Effective communication strategies can help to prevent medication errors and improve the quality of patient care.

2. True. Body movements or mannerisms can indicate one's feelings or psychological state of mind.

3. False. One of the most important things to remember about verbal communication is that "once it has been said, it can be taken back" because you can always explain why you said what you said. *One of the most important things to remember about verbal communication is that "once it has been said, it can't be taken back."*

4. False. When communicating using e-mail, it is acceptable to use all upper case letters because this makes the message clearer. *Internet "etiquette" also dictates that e-mail and business-related messages not be composed of all uppercase letters, to prevent the perception of shouting" or "scolding."*

5. True. Aggressive behavior, in which an individual displays an overbearing or intimidating attitude, can result in conflict and create a combative atmosphere and a perception of disrespect.

6. False. Open-ended questions are questions that can be answered with a simple "yes" or "no." *Close-ended questions are questions that can be answered with a simple "yes" or "no."*

7. False. Older patients generally have low general and health literacy skills. *Old age should not be confused with low general and health literacy skills. Assess all patients with regard to hearing, understanding, and general health literacy skills.*

8. False. Sensitivity to the cultural differences is not necessary because to be fair, everyone should receive the same treatment. *Sensitivity to the cultural differences in patient populations is necessary to help ensure effective communication.*

9. False. There is no excuse for patients to be hostile. *Patients are often coping with a number of personal issues and serious health conditions and concerns. Some patients are better able to cope with these challenges than others.*

10. True. Regardless of outward behaviors, patients need to feel that care and understanding is being extended to them.

Fill in the Blank Key

1. Judgmental
2. Close
3. The Health Insurance Portability and Accountability Act or HIPAA
4. Teamwork
5. Health literacy
6. Older
7. Patient-centered or pharmaceutical

8. Nonverbal

9. Empathy

10. Listening

Short Answer Key

1. Many scenarios may be described in answer to this question. Important points include:

   a. Professionalism.
   b. Care and respect.
   c. Assertive behavior.
   d. Active listening skills.
   e. Empathy.
   f. Appropriate body language.
   g. Appropriate physical distance and contact.

2. Close-ended questions are questions that can be answered with a simple "yes" or "no." An example of a close-ended question is, "Are you allergic to any medications?" Open-ended questions are questions that require a more elaborate response. An example of an open-ended question is, "What medications are you allergic to?" They can help verify or clarify understanding of information by requesting patients to elaborate on the concepts being discussed. A follow-up question may be needed to further elicit important information. If the patient indicates the presence of a medication allergy, an important follow-up question to ask would be, "Can you describe what happens when you take the medication?" The question, "What else are you allergic to?" would be asked until the patient verifies that no more allergies are present. Open-ended questions should be used to gather more in depth answers.

3. A judgmental response to the situation above could be viewed as devaluing the patient's concern, as in: "You seem to be the only one concerned about our ability to provide you with the correct medication quickly. All our other patients really love us and don't seem to care about the wait."

   An advice-giving response to the situation could be viewed as evidence that the technician thinks that the patient doesn't understand or hasn't thought through the comments; it might consist of the following statement: "You need to talk to the other patients who are waiting here. They will tell you that we know more about medicine and the prescription-filling process than you do."

A quizzing response to the situation could be viewed as evidence that the technician thinks the patient is confused or wrong; for example: "Think back to when you have picked up medication at other pharmacies. I don't believe that you have gotten it as quickly as we are going to give it to you."

A placating response to the situation above could be viewed as condescending, for example: "Oh, you shouldn't worry so much about the length of time. Just shop around for a while until it is ready, and try not to get yourself so worked up."

4. Various strategies can be used by technicians in the pharmacy to identify individuals who lack general and health literacy skills. These "red flags" include patients who decline when asked to read or fill out a form, explaining that they have "forgotten their glasses" or "have a headache." Patients lacking literacy skills may always bring family members or friends to fill out paperwork on their behalf and rarely look at prescription labels when discussing medication but only want to look at the medication itself. They may ask the questions contained in the patient information handouts and exhibit problems with medication adherence.

5. Pharmacy technicians can be effective members of the health care team by adopting the following behaviors:

   a. Cultivating trust and confidence among team members.
   b. Recognizing the contributions of all team members.
   c. Working with other team members to solve problems and develop ideas.
   d. Minimizing politics by respecting professional boundaries.
   e. Helping align the team around the objectives and priorities the members have in common.
   f. Establishing respect and appreciation among team members.
   g. Holding oneself and other team members to the same high standards.
   h. Putting the team's goals ahead of personal interests and goals.

Word Search Key

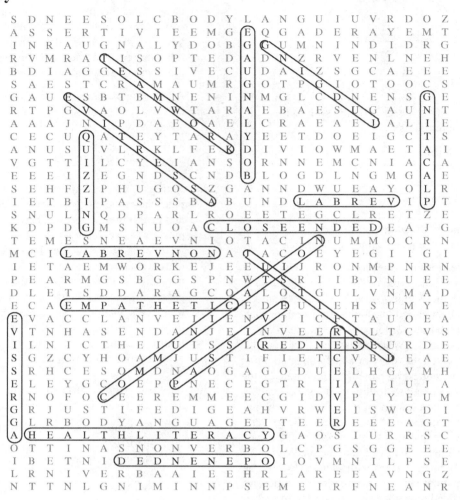

Chapter 9 Answer Keys

Multiple Choice Key

1. c. Cortex.

2. a. The central nervous system and the peripheral nervous system.

3. c. Pathophysiology.

4. c. Hypertension.

5. b. Heart, blood vessels, and blood.

6. b. The right atria and the right ventricle pump blood into the lungs.

7. d. Autonomic nervous system.

8. c. Coronary artery disease.

9. c. Both a and b.

10. a. Allows oxygen to be taken to cells in the body and carbon dioxide to be removed from the same cells.

11. b. 206

12. b. Smooth

13. d. All of the above.

14. d. Control the tear glands around the eye that produce tears to lubricate the eye.

15. a. Sclera/cornea.

16. d. Vestibular apparatus.

17. d. Antiseptics.

18. b. Epidermis and dermis.

19. d. Estrogen and progesterone.

20. d. All of the above.

Matching I Key

1. C. Alzheimer's disease

2. F. Attention deficit hyperactivity disorder

3. D. Mood disorders

4. B. Parkinson's disease

5. E. Psychotic disorders

6. A. Seizure disorders

Matching II Key

1. J. A state of unresponsiveness to a specific antigen or group of antigens to which a person is normally responsive.

2. D. The internal secretion of substances into the systemic circulation (bloodstream).

3. F. Reproductive organs—testes in the male and ovaries in the female.

4. G. Unhealthy function in an individual body system or an organ due to a disease.

5. A. A misdirected immune response that happens when the body attacks itself.

6. H. Waves of involuntary muscular contractions in the digestive tract.

7. I. The study of how living organisms function normally, including such processes as nutrition, movement, and reproduction.

8. E. Glands that have no ducts; their secretions are absorbed directly into the blood.

9. B. When the heart muscle is relaxed and the chambers are filling with blood; the pressure is at the lowest point in a normal heart.

10. C. The process whereby ingested food is broken up into smaller molecules by chemical or mechanical means.

True or False Key

1. True. The ability of the central and peripheral nervous systems to communicate with and regulate the function of organs in the body is possible through the release of neurotransmitters.

2. False. Alzheimer's disease is a condition where the myelin sheath is broken down, causing lesions on the nerves, problems with speech, difficulty swallowing, and muscle weakness. *These symptoms describe multiple sclerosis.*

3. False. The two most common mood disorders are anxiety and psychosis. *The two most common mood disorders are depression and bipolar disorder, also known as manic-depressive disorder.*

4. False. Acute pain typically lasts for months to years and may be accompanied by other symptoms such as sleep problems, lack of appetite, and depression. *Chronic pain typically lasts for months to years and may be accompanied by other symptoms such as sleep problems, lack of appetite, and depression.*

5. True. Common symptoms of schizophrenia include hallucinations (hearing or seeing things that are not real) and delusions (fixed beliefs that are false).

6. False. The white blood cells (leukocytes) are responsible for transporting oxygen to, and carbon dioxide away, from the cells of body tissues. *The red blood cells (erythrocytes) are responsible for transporting oxygen to, and carbon dioxide away, from the cells of body tissues.*

7. False. Two upper chambers are called the ventricles, which are found on the left and right sides of the heart; below them are the two atria. *Two upper chambers are called the atria, which are found on the left and right sides of the heart; below them are the two ventricles.*

8. True. Veins deliver blood *to* the heart, and arteries take blood *away* from the heart.

9. False. When the electrical activity of the heart is abnormal, a condition known as anemia develops. *When the electrical activity of the heart is abnormal, a condition known as an arrhythmia develops.*

10. True. The cause of a stroke can be a blood clot or a blood vessel that has ruptured.

11. False. Hypertension is a condition where a person is unable to cope with stressful events. *Hypertension occurs when the normal regulation of blood pressure is disrupted and the diastolic pressure remains chronically elevated—over 90 mmHg— and is accompanied by an increased systolic pressure of over 140 mm Hg.*

Part 2

12. False. Skeletal muscle is the primary muscle found in the internal organs of the body: stomach, intestines, glands, and blood vessels. *Smooth muscle is the primary muscle found in the internal organs of the body: stomach, intestines, glands, and blood vessels.*

13. False. Osteoarthritis is an inflammatory disease of the joints believed to be an autoimmune disease whereby the body produces specific proteins called antibodies that cause inflammation of a special membrane around the joints. *Rheumatoid arthritis is an inflammatory disease of the joints believed to be an autoimmune disease whereby the body produces specific proteins called antibodies that cause inflammation of a special membrane around the joints.*

14. True. Generally, problems within the endocrine system are due to one of two things: either too little or too much of a hormone is produced.

15. True. The organs of the immune system are connected with one another and with other organs of the body by a network of lymphatic vessels similar to blood vessels.

16. True. The ultimate goal of inflammation is to bring more help from the immune system to destroy the invaders, remove the dead cells, and begin the process of tissue healing and repair.

17. False. Drugs called antiarrhythmics are commonly used to treat and prevent allergies. *Drugs called antihistamines are commonly used to treat and prevent allergies.*

18. False. The pulmonary system terminates in single-layered cell structures called bronchioles, where the exchange of gases takes place between the lungs and the blood. *The pulmonary system terminates in single-layered cell structures called alveoli, where the exchange of gases takes place between the lungs and the blood.*

19. True. Chronic Obstructive Pulmonary Disease (COPD) includes two conditions known as emphysema and chronic obstructive bronchitis.

20. True. Actin and myosin are responsible for making a muscle contract and relax.

21. False. An individual suffering from hyperthyroidism can be treated with thyroid hormone replacement. *An individual suffering from hypothyroidism can be treated with thyroid hormone replacement.*

22. False. Diabetes insipidus is treated with insulin. *Diabetes insipidus is treated with vasopressin.*

Fill in the Blank Key

1. Anatomy
2. Physiology
3. Afferent
4. Somatic
5. Flight-or-fight
6. Four
7. Asthma
8. Osteoporosis
9. 1
10. 2
11. Immune
12. Conjunctivitis
13. Contact dermatitis
14. Eczema
15. Sexually transmitted diseases (STDs)
16. Benign prostatic hyperplasia (BPH)

Short Answer Key

1. See pages 189-191 in the *Manual for Pharmacy Technicians, 4th edition.*
2. See pages 169-172 in the *Manual for Pharmacy Technicians, 4th edition.*
3. See pages 173-178 in the *Manual for Pharmacy Technicians, 4th edition.*
4. See pages 183-185 in the *Manual for Pharmacy Technicians, 4th edition.*
5. See pages 185-188 in the *Manual for Pharmacy Technicians, 4th edition.*

Crossword Puzzle Key

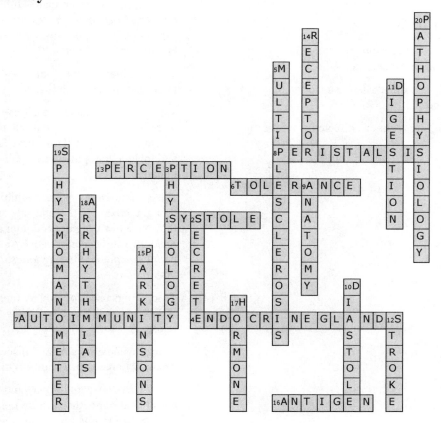

Chapter 10 Answer Keys

Multiple Choice Key

1. d. All of the above.

2. d. All of the above.

3. d. All of the above.

4. b. Suicidal thoughts or behavior.

5. c. Maintain function and quality of life.

6. a. Decreasing acetylcholine and increasing dopamine.

7. c. Memory impairment and behavioral changes.

8. d. Symptoms may include memory loss and confusion.

9. d. Maximize the amount of medications needed.

10. c. All of the above.

11. c. All of the above.

12. e. None of the above.

13. b. Reduce low density lipoprotein (LDL) levels and increase high density lipoprotein (HDL) levels.

14. e. None of the above.

15. d. ACE inhibitors can clear up bothersome dry coughs.

16. d. All of the above.

17. d. All of the above.

18. b. Acetylcholine blockers.

19. b. Known to cause thrush (fungus of the throat and mouth) in some patients.

20. a. There is little scientific evidence to show that they effectively aid in expectoration.

21. d. All of the above.

22. d. None of the above.

23. c. Using pain scales.

24. b. Can be given only by subcutaneous or intravenous injection.

25. a. Propylthiouracil (PTU).

26. c. Antihistamines have been shown to effectively shorten the duration of the common cold.

27. a. Used for rhinitis and other allergic or inflammatory conditions of the nose.

28. d. May be used in drug regimens directed at eradicating *H. pylori*.

29. d. All of the above.

30. d. All of the above.

Matching Key

1. G. Cyanocobalamin

2. H. Niacin (Nicotinic Acid)

3. E. Pantothenic Acid

4. F. Pyridoxine

5. A. Retinol

6. D. Riboflavin

7. C. Thiamine

8. B. Tocopherol

True or False Key

1. True. Antiepileptic agents should not be discontinued abruptly.

2. True. There may be differences in the bioavailability (extent of absorption) of the antiepileptic generics versus brand-name drugs, which may correlate to an increase in adverse effects/toxicities or an increase in seizure frequency.

3. False. Phenytoin is an injectable medication that is converted to fosphenytoin (Cerebyx) in the body. *Fosphenytoin (Cerebyx) is an injectable medication that is converted to phenytoin in the body.*

4. False. Phenytoin IV must only be mixed in dextrose. If phenytoin is mixed with normal saline, a precipitate will form. *Phenytoin IV must only be mixed in normal saline. If phenytoin is mixed with dextrose, a precipitate will form.*

5. True. The most common agents used in MS patients are those to prevent relapses and disease progression, and they have become known as the ABC therapy (Avonex, Betaseron, Copaxone).

6. False. The most common class of medications used for the treatment of migraines is Interferon-β-1b (Betaseron). *The most common class of medications used for the treatment of migraines is the serotonin 5-HT1 receptor agonists or the "triptans."*

7. True. Antidepressant medications are often used in the treatment of neuropathic pain.

8. True. The drugs used in the treatment of mood disorders work by altering the various chemicals, called neurotransmitters, found at the nerve junctions in the brain and include norepinephrine, epinephrine, serotonin, and dopamine.

9. False. Monoamine oxidase inhibitors (MAO-Is) are thought to be effective and safe antidepressants because they have few drug or food interactions. *MAO-Is are not typically used because they have drug-diet interactions with tyramine-containing foods and many drug-drug interactions.*

10. True. Drugs used for anxiety (anxiolytics) include SSRIs, benzodiazepines, SNRIs, TCAs, and buspirone (Buspar).

11. True. Psychosis is a mental disorder in which a person's capacity to recognize reality is distorted.

12. False. Benzodiazepines may and should be stopped abruptly at 6 months because they are habit forming. *Withdrawal symptoms can occur when benzodiazepines are taken for a long time and then abruptly stopped.*

13. False. The atypical antipsychotic agents have been shown to be more effective than the older agents. *The atypical antipsychotic agents have not been shown to be more effective than the older agents; however, they tend to have less EPS and may also have some mood-stabilizing effects because of their serotonergic properties.*

14. True. Omega-3 fatty acids (Lovaza), commonly found in fish oil, have been shown to reduce triglyceride levels in patients with very high triglycerides in their blood (hypertriglyceridemia).

15. True. The HMG-CoA reductase inhibitors are also known as "statins."

16. False. Loop diuretics are less potent diuretics and have fewer effects on electrolytes such as sodium, potassium, chloride, calcium, and magnesium than the thiazides. *Loop diuretics are more potent diuretics and may affect electrolytes such as sodium, potassium, chloride, calcium, and magnesium to a greater degree than the thiazides.*

17. True. ACE inhibitors may slow or prevent the development of kidney disease in diabetic patients and increase

survival, alleviate symptoms, and decrease hospitalization in patients with heart failure.

18. False. The ACE inhibitors have a –olol ending on the name. *The ACE inhibitors have a –pril ending on the name and beta blockers end with –olol.*

19. True. After 24 hours of continuous therapy, nitrates no longer work.

20. False. Asthma inhalers are meant to treat an acute attack (i.e., "quick-relief"). *Some inhalers are meant to prevent an attack (i.e., "controllers"), and some inhalers are used to treat an acute attack (i.e., "quick-relief").*

21. True. Patients with hypertension, heart disease, overactive thyroid, diabetes mellitus, or an enlarged prostate gland should use caution if taking decongestants.

22. True. Adequate calcium intake is essential for the prevention and treatment of osteoporosis.

23. True. All NSAIDs can cause serious bleeding and ulcers in the stomach.

24. True. All muscle relaxants cause sedation.

25. False. Opioid analgesics control pain, reduce inflammation, lower fever, and suppress cough and diarrhea. *Opioid analgesics do not reduce inflammation or lower fever.*

26. True. Insulin can be given only by subcutaneous or intravenous injection.

27. False. Oral hypoglycemic agents are used to lower blood sugar in Type 1 diabetes. *Oral hypoglycemic agents are used to lower blood sugar in Type 2 diabetes.*

28. True. Diseases of the thyroid gland include hypothyroidism (underproduction of thyroid hormone) and hyperthyroidism (overproduction of thyroid hormone).

29. False. Antihistamines often cause excitation, but a paradoxical reaction of drowsiness rather than excitation is sometimes seen in children and the elderly. *Antihistamines often cause drowsiness, but a paradoxical reaction of excitation rather than drowsiness is sometimes seen in children and the elderly.*

30. True. Since the antacid aluminum hydroxide commonly causes constipation and the antacid magnesium hydroxide commonly causes diarrhea, these antacids are combined to try to avoid either constipation or diarrhea.

31. False. When treating nausea and vomiting, OTC medications are generally used first before moving to prescription medications. *The antiemetic drug and route that are used depend on the cause and how often and how severe the nausea and vomiting are.*

32. False. Inflammatory bowel disease is usually controlled by the use of a single agent. *Goals of treatment include the resolution of abdominal pain, diarrhea, inflammation, and other symptoms. This is generally accomplished with the use of multiple medications.*

33. False. Diseases on or near the surface of the eye are most often treated with oral topical medications. *Diseases on or near the surface of the eye can often be treated with topical medications. Topical treatment of eye diseases is advantageous because the side effects that might occur with systemic (oral) medications can be avoided.*

34. True. Eye drops may have systemic effects. *Although ophthalmic drugs have low systemic absorption, ophthalmic beta-blockers can cause bronchoconstriction and slowed heart rate in some patients.*

35. False. Ophthalmic vasoconstrictors, or "decongestants," are commonly used to reduce redness in the eyes from minor irritations, are available over the counter for this purpose, and may be used indefinitely. *The over-the-counter products should not be used for more than 72 hours without consulting a physician.*

36. False. Topical ear treatments are commonly used for conditions involving the middle or inner ear. *Conditions involving the middle or inner ear require systemic treatment.*

37. True. Oral contraceptives are used to prevent pregnancy, to regulate menstruation, to treat endometriosis, to treat polycystic ovary syndrome, and to treat acne vulgaris.

38. False. A woman is considered to have infertility problems after attempting to conceive for over 3 years without success. *A woman is considered to have infertility problems after attempting to conceive for over 1 year without success.*

39. False. Benign prostatic hypertrophy (BPH) is a noncancerous enlargement of the prostate gland that develops in older men and women. *Benign prostatic hypertrophy only affects men.*

40. True. The severity, site, and source of infection; characteristics of the antibiotic; and characteristics of the patient are all considered when an antibiotic is selected.

41. True. Penicillin allergies are estimated to occur in 5 to 8% of the population and can be fatal.

42. False. Patients who are allergic to penicillin should not take the macrolides. *Patients who are allergic to penicillin can safely take the macrolides.*

43. False. Fluoroquinolones may be used in the general population for treatment of urinary tract infections, re-

spiratory infections, and gastrointestinal infections and as single-dose therapy for some sexually transmitted diseases. *Fluoroquinolones are contraindicated in pregnant women and children because of possible effects on bone growth.*

44. False. Vancomycin is usually given intravenously or orally for treatment of systemic infections. *Oral vancomycin is not absorbed well enough to treat systemic infections.*

45. True. The Centers for Disease Control and Prevention, an agency of the U.S. Government, has published guidelines for the prevention and treatment of TB.

46. False. Herpes simplex virus causes the very painful symptoms of shingles and the potentially serious cases of chicken pox in people with weakened immune systems (e.g., children with leukemia). *Herpes zoster causes the very painful symptoms of shingles and the potentially serious cases of chicken pox in people with weakened immune systems (e.g., children with leukemia).*

47. False. Anti-HIV antivirals have been developed that may be effectively used as monotherapy. *Anti-HIV antivirals work on different enzymes involved with replication of the virus. Because they work on different enzymes, a combination of drugs from different classes enhances their effectiveness and delays the emergence of resistant strains of HIV.*

48. True. Liposomal amphotericin B formulations are less toxic to the kidneys and cause fewer infusion-related adverse events when compared with conventional amphotericin.

49. False. Colony-stimulating factors are used to increase red blood cells. *Colony-stimulating factors are used to increase white blood cells. A decrease in white blood cells may occur due to antineoplastic therapy or in HIV/AIDS.*

50. True. Because anticoagulants slow clot formation, the main concern with anticoagulant therapy is excessive bleeding.

Fill in the Blank Key

1. Anticonvulsants

2. Status epilepticus

3. Triptans

4. Neuropathic

5. Black box warnings

6. Tricyclic

7. Bipolar

8. Psychosis

9. Amnesia

10. Diuretics

11. Nitrates

12. Corticosteroids

13. Osteoporosis

14. Penicillin

15. Aminoglycoside

16. Vancomycin

17. Herpes simplex

18. Warfarin (Coumadin)

19. K

20. Potassium

Short Answer Key

1. See pages 205-218 in the *Manual for Pharmacy Technicians, 4th edition.*

2. See pages 218-224 in the *Manual for Pharmacy Technicians, 4th edition.*

3. See pages 224-228 in the *Manual for Pharmacy Technicians, 4th edition.*

4. See pages 228-232 in the *Manual for Pharmacy Technicians, 4th edition.*

5. See pages 232-235 in the *Manual for Pharmacy Technicians, 4th edition.*

6. See pages 235-236 in the *Manual for Pharmacy Technicians, 4th edition.*

7. See pages 236-240 in the *Manual for Pharmacy Technicians, 4th edition.*

8. See pages 240-241 in the *Manual for Pharmacy Technicians, 4th edition.*

9. See pages 241-245 in the *Manual for Pharmacy Technicians, 4th edition.*

10. See pages 249-255 in the *Manual for Pharmacy Technicians, 4th edition.*

11. See pages 257-260 in the *Manual for Pharmacy Technicians, 4th edition.*

Alphabet Soup Key

a.   USAN: United States Adopted Names Council

b.   PD: Parkinson's Disease

c.   MS: Multiple Sclerosis

d.   OTC: Over the Counter

e.   SSRIs: Selective Serotonin Reuptake Inhibitors

f.   SNRIs: Serotonin-Norepinephrine Reuptake Inhibitors

g.   MAOIs: Monoamine Oxidase Inhibitors

h.   TCAs: Tricyclic Antidepressants

i.   OCD: Obsessive Compulsive Disorder

j.   IM: Intramuscular

k.   EPS: Extrapyramidal Symptoms

l.   ADHD: Attention Deficit Hyperactivity Disorder

m.   LDL: Low Density Lipoprotein

n.   HDL: High Density Lipoprotein

o.   TG: Triglycerides

p.   CAD: Coronary Artery Disease

q.   ACE inhibitors: Angiotensin-Converting Enzyme Inhibitors

r.   ARBs: Angiotensin Receptor Blockers

s.   COPD: Chronic Obstructive Pulmonary Disease

t.   MDI: Metered-Dose Inhaler

u.   NSAIDs: Nonsteroidal Anti-Inflammatory Drugs

v.   PTU: Propylthiouracil

w.   MMR: Measles-Mumps-Rubella

x.   DTaP: Diphtheria-Tetanus-Pertussis

y.   HPV: Human Papillomavirus

z.   PUD: Peptic Ulcer Disease

aa.   GERD: Gastroesophageal Reflux Disease

bb.   MOM: Milk of Magnesia

cc.   IBD: Inflammatory Bowel Disease

dd.   SPF: Sun Protection Factor

ee.   FSH: Follicle-Stimulating Hormone

ff.   hMG: Human Menopausal Gonadotropin

gg.   HCG: Human Chorionic Gonadotropin

hh.   HRT: Hormone Replacement Therapy

ii.   BPH: Benign Prostatic Hypertrophy

jj.   ED: Erectile Dysfunction

kk.   VRE: Vancomycin-Resistant Enterococci

ll.   TB: Tuberculosis

mm.   HIV: Human Immunodeficiency Virus

nn.   RSV: Respiratory Syncytial Virus

oo.   CMV: Cytomegalovirus

pp.   CSF: Colony-Stimulating Factor

qq.   EPO: Erythropoietin Alfa

rr.   HIT: Heparin-Induced Thrombocytopenia

ss.   UFH: Unfractionated Heparin

tt.   LMWHs: Low-Molecular Weight Heparins

uu.   DVT: Deep Vein Thrombosis

vv.   AMI: Acute Myocardial Infarction

ww.   RDA: Recommended Dietary Allowance

xx.   CAM: Complementary and Alternative Medicine

Chapter 11 Answer Keys

Multiple Choice Key

1.   d. All of the above.

2.   d. Absorption, distribution, metabolism, excretion.

3.   d. All of the above.

4.   b. Inhalation.

5.   d. All of the above.

6.   b. The movement of a drug through the body.

7.   a. Are 100% bioavailable.

8.   d. All of the above.

9.   d. All of the above.

10.   b. Kidneys.

Matching Key

1.   M. A breakdown product of a medication that has undergone metabolism.

2.   E. A group of enzymes that metabolize drugs.

3.   K. A larger first dose given to quickly achieve a high drug concentration in the body.

4. A. The process of medication entering the bloodstream or systemic circulation.

5. P. The blood level at which most patients receive a medication's desired effect with minimal side effects.

6. F. The breakdown of medication from its original solid formulation.

7. L. The breakdown of medication in the body.

8. G. The dissolving of medication into solution, usually in the stomach and intestinal tract.

9. Q. The extent of a medication's outreach to various tissues and spaces throughout the body.

10. H. The impact of a drug or food product on the amount or activity of another drug in the body.

11. I. The metabolism (breaking down) of orally ingested medications by the liver and small intestine before they reach the main bloodstream.

12. B. The percentage of an administered dose of a medication that reaches the bloodstream.

13. C. The study of the manufacture of medications for effective delivery into the body.

14. O. The study of the movement of a drug through the body during the following phases: absorption, distribution, metabolism, and excretion.

15. N. The study of the relationship between the concentration of a drug in the body and the response or outcome observed or measured in a patient.

16. J. The time that it takes for 50% of a drug to be eliminated from the body.

17. D. The total removal of a drug via metabolism and/or excretion.

True or False Key

1. False. Disintegration is the dissolving of medication into solution, usually in the stomach and intestinal tract. *Dissolution is the dissolving of medication into solution, usually in the stomach and intestinal tract.*

2. False. Some medications that are administered intravenously are metabolized (broken down) before they reach the main bloodstream, which is referred to as first-pass metabolism. *This occurs with some medications administered orally.*

3. False. The medication bound to blood proteins is active and exerts its pharmacologic effect while it is bound to the protein. *The medication bound to blood proteins is inactive and does not exert any pharmacologic effect until it is released from the protein.*

4. True. The therapeutic level for medications is the level at which most patients receive the desired effect with minimal side effects.

5. False. In general, medications with a large volume of distribution will have a higher blood concentration, whereas medications with a small volume of distribution will have a lower blood concentration. *Medications with a large volume of distribution will have a lower blood concentration, whereas medications with a small volume of distribution will have a higher blood concentration.*

6. True. If a medication is widely distributed throughout the body and the prescriber wants the medication to start working quickly, sometimes a loading dose of the medication will be given to more quickly achieve a higher drug concentration in the body.

7. False. Most medications require a loading dose. *Most medications do not require a loading dose.*

8. False. Most drug metabolism occurs in the kidneys, although significant metabolism can occur in the small intestine. *Most drug metabolism occurs in the liver, although significant metabolism can occur in the small intestine.*

9. True. The most common enzymes that metabolize drugs belong to a family of enzymes called the cytochrome P450 (CYP) system.

10. True. A "pro-drug" is where a drug is administered in an inactive form, which is metabolized or converted to the active component.

Fill in the Blank Key

1. Biopharmaceutics

2. Absorption

3. Dissolution

4. Bioavailability

5. Albumin

6. Metabolism

7. Excretion

8. Drug interaction

9. Creatinine

10. Agonists

11. Half-life

Short Answer Key

1. The pharmacy technician is often the first person in the pharmacy to handle a patient's medication, often filling multiple prescriptions for a single patient. Thus, the pharmacy technician who prepares prescriptions for dispensing should have a basic understanding of biopharmaceutics, pharmacokinetics, and pharmacodynamics, which collectively describe how a particular medication is prepared, is handled by the body, and affects the body. Having this understanding can help avoid unwanted (adverse) drug events because the complex interactions of many medications is a risk factor for adverse drug events—especially in older individuals and certain other patient populations, as will be described in more detail in this chapter. For example, a prescriber may write that a particular prescription medication should be crushed before being taken; however, a knowledgeable pharmacy technician may know crushing that particular medication results in loss of the slow-release properties of the drug. Likewise, a pharmacy technician knowledgeable about the absorption of a particular medication may know that it should not be taken with certain other medications or dietary agents that could affect its absorption. An understanding of basic biopharmaceutical, pharmacokinetic, and pharmacodynamic principles can aid the clinician in appropriately monitoring medication therapy, and the pharmacy technician can aid the pharmacist in such surveillance.

2. See pages 268 and 272–276 of the *Manual for Pharmacy Technicians, 4th edition.*

3. Drugs (and some foods) can compete with other drugs for metabolism within the system or alter the metabolic system altogether, resulting in drug interactions. A drug interaction is defined as the impact of a drug or food product on the amount or activity of another drug in the body. This drug-drug (or drug-food) interaction can result in enhanced, reduced, or new activity of the drug in the body. The most common cause of drug interactions is altered drug metabolism in the liver. For example, some medications, foods, and herbal products can inhibit (or slow down) enzyme activity, which results in reduced drug metabolism of other medications. Conversely, some drugs can induce (or speed up) the metabolism of other medications. These two mechanisms are the most common forms of drug interactions. Thus, knowing the metabolic effects of each medication dispensed to a patient can help determine if a drug interaction is likely to occur.

4. Pharmacodynamics refers to the study of the relationship between the concentration of a drug in the body and the response or outcome observed or measured in a patient. Examples of pharmacodynamic responses include an increase in bone mass with a bisphosphonate used for osteoporosis, a decrease in blood pressure with an antihypertensive agent, and a decrease in blood glucose with a sulfonylurea used in the management of diabetes.

5. For a pharmacologic effect to occur, a drug needs to be absorbed into the systemic circulation and travel to its intended site of action, or target organ, as described earlier. Next, it needs to bind to a specific receptor, like a key fitting into a lock. A receptor is a protein that is embedded on the surface of the cell and that allows communication between the outside and the inside of the cell. Once the drug binds to the receptor, this triggers a cascade of events that leads to the drug's response. The time that it takes to detect a drug's response, whether it be very rapid or delayed, is related to the drug-receptor binding process and to any subsequent chemical reactions that take place inside the target cell or organ. By binding to the receptor, medications can either promote or block the signal that would ordinarily be generated by binding of the normally occurring substance to the receptor. Medications that augment or enhance a signal normally communicated in a cell are called agonists. Medications that block the transmission of a signal normally communicated in a cell are called antagonists. The drug-receptor complex forms the basis of medication effects on the body. This drug-receptor interaction is what makes medications work.

Part **2**

Word Search Key

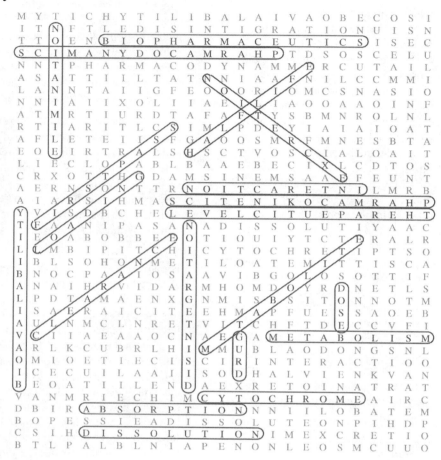

Chapter 12 Answer Keys

Multiple Choice Key

1. a. Water, alcohol, glycerin, and mineral oil.

2. d. All of the above.

3. d. All of the above.

4. a. Alcohol can have undesired interactions with other medications the patients may be taking.

5. d. All of the above.

6. d. All of the above.

7. d. None of the above.

8. d. All of the above.

9. e. None of the above.

10. d. All of the above.

Matching Key

1. V. Applied to skin or mucous membranes

2. E. By way of the intestine

3. F. Bypassing the gastrointestinal tract

4. P. Immediately under the skin (SubQ, SC, SQ)

5. B. Inside the cheek

6. H. Into a joint (IA)

   Note that IA stands for intra-articular and intra-arterial—one of the dangers of using abbreviations!

7. L. Into a vein (IV)

8. G. Into an artery (IA)

   Note that IA stands for intra-articular and intra-arterial—one of the dangers of using abbreviations!

9. S. Into the ear

10. O. Into the eye

11. R. Into the eye

12. I. Into the heart muscle (IC)

13. Q. Into the nose

14. K. Into the space around the spinal cord

15. J. Into the top layers of the skin (ID)

16. N. Into the urinary bladder

17. M. Into the ventricles, or cavities, of the brain

18. U. Through the anus

19. A. Through the mouth (PO)

20. T. Through the skin

21. W. Through the skin

22. D. Under the gums

23. C. Under the tongue (SL)

True or False Key

1. True. For a systemic effect to take place, absorption of the medication must occur.

2. False. Liquid medications are always solutions. *The medication can be dissolved in the vehicle (solution) or can be present as very fine solid particles that are suspended, or floating, in the vehicle.*

3. False. All liquid medications may be made palatable by adding flavors and sweetening agents. *Even with such sweetening or flavoring, the taste of some liquid medications may remain unpleasant.*

4. True. Aqueous solutions can be injected into the bloodstream.

5. False. Solid medication dosage forms are usually faster-acting than liquid medication dosage forms. *Oral liquid medication dosage forms are usually faster-acting than solid medication dosage forms.*

6. False. Medications may be absorbed into the bloodstream as very small particles suspended in an aqueous vehicle. *Medications are absorbed into the bloodstream in a dissolved state.*

7. False. Like gargles, mouthwashes should be swallowed. *Like gargles, mouthwashes should not be swallowed.*

8. False. Simple syrup contains sucrose, flavoring, and water. *Simple syrup contains only sucrose and water.*

9. False. The only uses for enemas are to relieve severe constipation or to clean the large bowel before surgery. *Enemas are solutions that are inserted into the rectum to empty the lower intestinal tract or to treat diseases of that area.*

10. True. Elixirs and spirits are examples of hydroalcoholic solutions.

11. True. Elixirs should be avoided by alcoholics.

12. True. Tablets that are enteric coated should not be crushed, chewed, or cut.

13. True. Suppositories may treat local conditions in the immediate area of administration or may exert systemic effects elsewhere.

14. True. If it seems necessary to crush, chew, or cut an extended-release product, an immediate-release formulation of the same drug should be used instead.

15. False. Continuous infusions may be given by IV push. *Boluses are given by IV push.*

Fill in the Blank Key

1. Local

2. Systemic

3. Tinctures

4. Fluidextracts

5. Emulsions

6. Effervescent

7. Granule

8. Suspensions

9. Mucilages

10. Buccal

11. PO

12. Parenteral

Part **2**

Short Answer Key

1. Advantages:

   • Oral liquid medication dosage forms are usually faster-acting than solid medication dosage forms. Medications are absorbed into the bloodstream in a dissolved state. The medication in a liquid medication dosage form is either already dissolved or is present in small particles which then dissolve in fluids in the gastrointestinal tract, so the medication can be readily absorbed into the bloodstream. In contrast, tablets must first dissolve in the stomach (or other place where they may be administered such as the vagina) before they can be absorbed, so it takes more time for the medication to be absorbed and to act.

   • For patients who have difficulty swallowing, oral liquid medications may be easier to take than oral solid medication dosage forms.

   • Liquid doses have more flexibility than some other dosage forms because liquid medications are usually dispensed in bulk containers rather than distinct dosage units. For example, a liquid medication contains 500 mg of a drug in 10 mL of liquid. The same medication is also available in 500-mg tablets. To take a 600-mg dose of the liquid medication, a patient would simply need to measure out 12 mL of liquid. However, to take a 600-mg dose of the tablet, the patient would need to take 1.2 tablets, which would be difficult.

   • Liquid medications may be used where solid medication dosage forms are not practical to administer. For example, medications that need to be placed directly into the ears or eyes can be administered more easily as a liquid than as a solid.

   Disadvantages:

   • Often, liquid medication dosage forms have shorter times to expiration than other dosage forms.

   • Many drugs have an unpleasant taste as the drug dissolves or is chewed into small particles. Drug particles are already present in oral liquid medications and come in contact with the taste buds of the tongue. People often find the taste or sensation of these drug particles unpleasant. Sweeteners and flavoring agents are necessary to make these liquid medications taste better. Even with such sweetening or flavoring, the taste of some liquid medications may remain unpleasant. Tablets and capsules, on the other hand, are often coated and can be swallowed quickly to avoid contact with the taste buds.

   • Patients sometimes find liquid medications inconvenient because they may be spilled, require careful measuring before administration, or have special storage or handling requirements such as refrigeration or shaking before use.

2. In most emulsions, the two liquids are oil and water. An oil-in-water (O/W) emulsion consists of small oil droplets scattered throughout water. O/W emulsions are desirable for oral use for several reasons. Unpleasant oily medications are broken into small particles and dispersed throughout a sweetened, flavored aqueous vehicle. These small particles are carried past the taste buds and swallowed without the patient tasting the oily medication. The small particle size increases medication absorption from the stomach and small intestine into the bloodstream. One formulation of cyclosporine (Neoral), a medication used to prevent rejection of transplanted organs, is such an example.

   In water-in-oil (W/O) emulsions, water droplets are spread throughout the oil. W/O emulsions are often used on unbroken skin. They spread more evenly than O/W emulsions because the natural oils of the skin mix with the external oil phase of the emulsion. They soften the skin better because they hold moisture and are not easily washed off with water. However, they have a heavy, greasy feel and may stain clothing.

   The choice of O/W or W/O emulsion for preparations applied to the skin depends on several factors. As an example, medications that are irritating to the skin feel better when applied as small particles in the internal phase. The external phase keeps them from directly contacting and irritating the skin. O/W emulsions may be more desirable in some cases because they are water-washable and do not stain. They feel lighter and nongreasy and have an advantage when the emulsion is to be applied to a hairy part of the body such as the scalp.

3. These inactive, or inert, ingredients (e.g., binders, diluents, lubricants, colorants) are necessary for the manufacturing process or to make the tablet more effective (e.g., disintegrators). Binders hold the compressed tablet together and keep it from crumbling. Diluents are fillers that are added to the active medication to make the tablet a practical size. Lubricants help in the removal of the tablet from the die punch. Colorants add color to the product. Disintegrators help the tablet break apart so it can dissolve more quickly in the stomach, in the small intestine, or elsewhere in the body. Compressed tablets may have a sugar, film, or enteric coating on the outside. Sugar coating or film coating may be used to mask foul-tasting or foul-smelling drugs, to add color

to the tablet, or to protect the drug from exposure to air and humidity. A film coating coats the tablet with a hard shell to make it sturdier and easier to swallow. Enteric-coated oral tablets have a coating that protects the lining of the stomach from irritation by the drug. The coating delays the dissolution of the tablet as it passes through the stomach and into the small intestine.

4. The primary types of ointment bases are oleaginous, anhydrous, emulsion, and water-soluble. Oleaginous, or hydrocarbon, bases are emollients that soothe the skin or mucous membranes. They are occlusive (provide a barrier) and protect the skin or mucous membrane from the air. They are hydrophobic (repel water), so they do not wash off with water and they feel greasy to the touch. Oleaginous bases are used mainly for their lubricating effect because they do not allow moisture to escape from the skin, do not dry out, and remain on the skin for a long time. Vaseline petroleum jelly is an example of an oleaginous base.

Anhydrous, or absorption, bases contain no water and are similar to oleaginous bases, but they absorb water instead of repelling it. They also soften skin, but not to the same degree as the oleaginous bases. Anhydrous bases absorb aqueous, or water-based, drugs. Anhydrous lanolin and cold cream are widely used anhydrous bases.

Emulsion bases may be water-in-oil (W/O) or oil-in-water (O/W). The W/O emulsion bases are emollient, occlusive, and greasy. They contain water, and some may be able to absorb additional water. Lanolin, mentioned above as an anhydrous base, and cold cream are considered to be W/O emulsions when water is added to them. Emulsion bases of the O/W type, or water-washable bases, are quite different. They are nongreasy and readily wash off with water. They are nonocclusive and may be diluted, or thinned, with the addition of water. In certain skin conditions, O/W emulsion bases are used to absorb watery discharge or to help the skin absorb certain medications.

Water-soluble bases are nongreasy, nonocclusive, and water-washable. They do not contain any fats and usually do not contain any water. Nonaqueous or solid medications are added to this type of ointment base. Polyethylene glycol ointment is one such base. Ointment bases are chosen primarily on the basis of the characteristics described above. A W/O emulsion base may be used if a liquid medication is to be added to the ointment. Some medications may be more stable or more readily absorbed by the skin when delivered in a particular type of ointment base. The softening or drying characteristics of the ointment base may also influence the choice of a base. For instance, a nongreasy ointment base may be chosen if the ointment is to be applied to the face, because a greasy base may leave an unpleasant feeling.

5. Extended-release dosage forms offer several advantages:

- They deliver medication in a slow, controlled, and consistent manner so the patient absorbs the same amount of medication throughout a given time period.

- The risk of drug side effects is reduced because the medication is delivered in smaller amounts over a long period of time rather than all at once.

- Patients may need to take the medication less frequently, perhaps only once or twice a day, or even as infrequently as once a week, once a month, or even longer.

- Patients are more likely to take their medications properly, and are less likely to experience side effects if they can take them less often.

- The daily medication cost to patients may be decreased. Although extended-release products may be more expensive on a per-dose basis, the total daily cost may be less because the patient takes fewer doses overall.

There are disadvantages to extended-release dosage forms:

- There may be a delay between the time the patient takes the medication and the time it takes effect. Therefore, extended-release products are not helpful in situations where an immediate effect is required.

- If a patient does experience a side effect, it may take some time for the effect to dissipate because some of the medication may remain in the body.

- Most extended-release products cannot be cut, crushed, or chewed. This may limit the situations in which the product may be used.

- The medication may be more expensive than an immediate-release product.

Alphabet Soup Key

a. CD: Controlled-Diffusion

b. CR: Controlled-Release, Continuous-Release

c. CRT: Controlled-Release Tablet

d. LA: Long-Acting

e. SA: Sustained-Action

f. SR: Sustained-Release, Slow-Release

g. TD: Time-Delay

h. TR: Time-Release

i. XL: Extra-Long

j. XR: Extended-Release

Crossword Puzzle Key

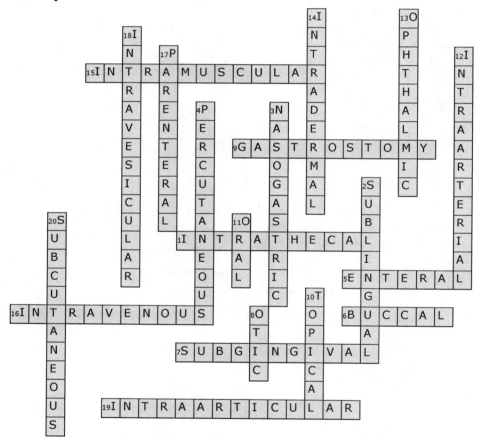

Chapter 13 Answer Keys

Multiple Choice Key

1. d. All of the above.

2. d. All of the above.

3. e. All of the above.

4. a. Check to see that the order makes sense for the patient by checking the order against the patient profile. *If an incorrect sticker is applied to an order, it will contain the wrong patient name as well as the wrong account number and the wrong medical record number.*

5. e. All of the above.

6. e. None of the above. *Standardized schedules of drug administration are usually based on therapeutic issues, nursing and pharmacy efficiency, or coordination of services.*

7. c. All of the above.

8. d. All of the above.

9. c. Aminoglycoside dosing and monitoring.

10. d. All of the above.

Matching Key

1. A,B. Patient name

2. A. Patient account number

3. A. Patient birth date

4. A. Patient allergies

5. B. Brand drug name

6. A,B. Route of administration

7. A,B. Dosage form

8. A,B. Dose/strength

9. A,B. Frequency and duration of administration (if duration is pertinent; may be open-ended)

10. C. Indication for use of the medication (Neither— unfortunately the indication for use is not required but would be very helpful in both instances.)

11. A,B. Other instructions for the person administering the medication, such as whether it should be given with food or on an empty stomach

12. C. Prescriber's name/signature and credentials

13. A. Date the order was written

14. C. Time the order was written (Neither—unfortunately the indication for use is not required but would be very helpful in both instances.)

15. A. Sex

16. A. Height and weight

17. C. Lab values such as serum creatinine

18. A. Room and bed number

19. B. Quantity to be dispensed

20. B. Number of refills to be allowed

21. C. Substitution authority or refusal

22. C. DEA number for controlled medications

True or False Key

1. False. If information is missing from a medication order or an order is unclear, most clarifications can be handled by the pharmacy technician. *Most clarifications must involve the pharmacist.*

2. True. An order for phenylephrine, a medication used intravenously to maintain blood pressure in critically ill patients, would usually receive priority over an order for an orally administered vitamin.

3. True. Medications ordered for the initial treatment of pain, fever, or nausea and vomiting are generally high priority because of the desire to relieve the patient's discomfort.

4. False. A patient's account number never changes, but medical record numbers change every time a patient is admitted to an institution. *A patient's medical record number never changes, but account numbers change every time a patient is admitted to an institution.*

5. False. It is recommended that prescribers order drug products by brand name instead of generic name. *It is recommended that prescribers order drug products by generic name instead of brand name.*

6. True. Default time schedules may differ on some specialized nursing units.

7. True. The last step in the order entry process is generally an acceptance (also called verification or validation) function in which the pharmacist verifies that the order is correctly entered for the right patient and is clinically appropriate.

8. False. If an inpatient is taking his medications brought in from home, there is no need to enter these medications into the computer system since the patient will not be charged for the medications. *It is important for the*

medications to show up on the MAR and in the patient profile so that all caregivers are aware that the patient is receiving the medication. There is also a legal record that the doses were administered, so these medications must be entered into the computer system.

9. False. With CPOE, it is not necessary for a pharmacist to review and verify the order before the medication is dispensed because the physician has entered the order. *With CPOE, a pharmacist still reviews and verifies the order before the medication is dispensed.*

10. False. In all states, when a prescriber signs his or her name over the DAW signature line, the medication must be dispensed as written. *Depending on state law, signatures may or may not be valid. Some states do not accept preprinted prescription blanks, and the prescriber must write "DAW."*

11. False. In the outpatient setting, prescriptions are always filled in the order in which they are presented to the pharmacy, and many pharmacies use some type of "take-a-number" system to be entirely fair. *Some common-sense judgment does apply in the outpatient setting. For example, regardless of the order in which they were presented, prescriptions for customers who are waiting are generally filled before prescriptions to be mailed the next day.*

12. False. As long as the correct drug is selected regarding medication name and strength, it is not necessary to match the NDC number with the product dispensed, especially when generic products are used. *It is necessary to match the NDC number with the product dispensed.*

13. False. Unlike inpatient pharmacies, there are no formulary issues in the outpatient setting. *Outpatient dispensing may be governed by numerous formularies, because each third-party payer has the option of identifying a formulary for its patients.*

14. True. A pharmacist check is legally required in most cases, and must occur before any drug is dispensed to a patient care area.

Fill in the Blank Key

1. Medication order

2. Prescription

3. CPOE

4. MAR

5. Tall man lettering

6. Central

7. Bar codes

8. Adjudication

9. Auxiliary

10. Mnemonic

Short Answer Key

1. Ideally, every medication order contains the following elements:

   - Patient name, hospital identification number, and room/bed location

   - Generic drug name (It is recommended that generic drug names be used, and many institutions have policies to this effect.)

   - Brand drug name (if a specific product is required)

   - Route of administration (With some orders, the site of administration should also be specified.)

   - Dosage form

   - Dose/strength

   - Frequency and duration of administration (if duration is pertinent; may be open-ended)

   - Rate and time of administration, if applicable

   - Indication for use of the medication

   - Other instructions for the person administering the medication such as whether it should be given with food or on an empty stomach

   - Prescriber's name/signature and credentials (Some hospitals require a printed name, physician number, or pager number in addition to the signature, to assist with identification.)

   - Signature and credentials of person writing the order, if other than prescriber

   - Date and time of the order

2. Technicians can prioritize orders by evaluating the route, time of administration, type of drug, intended use of the drug, and patient-specific circumstances. For example, an order for phenylephrine, a medication used intravenously to maintain blood pressure in critically ill patients, would usually receive priority over an order for an orally administered stool softener. Remember to think of patient needs first. Some orders are designated as STAT, which indicates an urgent need. A prescriber may also designate that a medication is to be started "now" or "ASAP" (as soon as possible), or simply state

"start today" or "start this morning." It is also necessary to consider whether a medication might already have been started prior to the pharmacy's receipt of the order—a first dose of an antibiotic administered in the emergency room prior to the patient's admission, for example. If no apparent urgency or specific time is denoted in the order, it may receive a lower priority.

Most pharmacies designate a standard amount of time it should take to process and deliver an order. A typical turnaround time for filling an order in an institutional setting might be 15 minutes for a STAT order and 1 hour for a routine order. If no specific designation about the urgency of a medication is given in the body of the order, technicians can use critical thinking skills to prioritize orders. Most of the decisions involved in prioritizing orders require some basic knowledge of the drugs and common sense. It is also helpful for technicians to be familiar with their hospital's specific policies regarding prioritization of orders. Some hospitals, for example, treat all orders from a particular unit—such as an intensive care unit—as urgent. Many hospitals have designated administration times for certain drugs (e.g., warfarin) that may alter prioritization of the order depending on the time the order is received. Policies vary by pharmacy, and technicians need to become familiar with the system of prioritization used at their institution.

3. Inpatient order entry usually proceeds as follows:

   a. Enter the patient's name or account number, and verify the patient.

   b. Compare the order to the patient profile in detail.

   c. Enter the drug.

   d. Verify the dose.

   e. Enter the administration schedule.

   f. Enter any comments in the clinical comments field.

   g. Verify the prescriber name.

   h. Fill and label the medication.

4. The following information is generally found in the hospital pharmacy's patient profile, although system capabilities may limit access to some components:

   • Patient name and identification numbers

   • Date of birth or age

   • Sex

   • Height and weight

   • Lab values such as serum creatinine

   • Admitting and secondary diagnoses (e.g., pregnancy, lactation status)

   • Room and bed number

   • Names of admitting and consulting physicians

   • Allergies

   • Medication history (current and discontinued medications; medications from a previous admission, if applicable)

   • Special considerations (e.g., foreign language, disability)

   • Clinical comments (e.g., therapeutic monitoring, counseling notes)

5. A fully implemented decentralized system would work something like this:

   a. An order is received in the pharmacy and is entered into the pharmacy computer system.

   b. Once order entry is completed, a computer interface sends the information to the automation device, effectively "releasing" the medication for use for a specific patient.

   c. The nurse goes to the machine and keys in the patient's name and the drug name, and the appropriate location in the device "unlocks" so that the medication can be removed.

   d. For continuing medications (e.g., a tid medication), the nurse goes back to the device at designated times (standard administration times) throughout the day and removes the medication for administration to the patient.

   e. When it is time to restock the machine, the technician prints a batch restock report that is filled by a technician and then checked by a pharmacist. The technician then makes a delivery to each unit and restocks the medications into the machines. Some devices allow for bar code verification of the medication to ensure that the correct medication goes to the correct bin.

Alphabet Soup Key

   a. CPOE: Computer Physician Order Entry

   b. MAR: Medication Administration Record

   c. eMAR: Electronic Medication Administration Record

   c. STAT: Immediately (from statim)

   e. ASAP: As Soon As Possible

f. QA: Quality Assurance

g. DAW: Dispense as Written

h. DNS: Do Not Substitute

i. NDC: National Drug Code

j. DEA: Drug Enforcement Agency

Chapter 14 Answer Keys

Multiple Choice Key

1. b. Convert to common denominators, add the numerators, reduce to the simplest fractions or mixed numbers.

2. b. Multiply the denominators, multiply the numerators, express answer as a fraction and simplify.

3. c. per 100.

4. d. Meter (distance), liter (volume), gram (mass).

5. c. All of the above.

6. d. All of the above.

7. b. There is one formula that is used to calculate BSA.

8. c. 20 drops.

9. c. Weight in volume (w/v) or grams of drug per 100 mL of mixture.

10. d. g per mL.

Matching Key

1. M. A combination of two ratios with the same units; a statement of equality between two ratios

2. C. A French system of mass that includes ounces and pounds

3. D. A measure of body fat based on height and weight used to determine if a patient is underweight, of normal weight, overweight, or obese

4. H. A part of a whole number used to express quantities less than one or quantities between two whole numbers

5. O. A ratio expressed as 1:something, where the units are g per mL. The concentrations of weak solutions such as 1:1000 or 1:10,000 epinephrine are sometimes expressed this way

6. N. A representation of the relationship between two items

7. I. A system of measurement commonly used in cooking, including the teaspoon, the tablespoon, and the cup

8. B. A system of measurement originally developed in Greece for use by physicians and pharmacists but now largely replaced by the metric system

9. A. A way to help determine how many parts of each strength should be mixed together to prepare the desired strength

10. J. An estimate of how much a patient should weigh based on his or her height and gender; expressed in kg

11. F. The time a specific amount of medication will last

12. G. The bottom number of a fraction, representing the total number of parts

13. K. The most widely used and accepted system of measurement in the world; based on multiples of ten

14. L. The top number of a fraction, representing the number of parts present

15. E. The total surface area of the body, taking the patient's weight and height into account and expressed in m2

True or False Key

1. False. Numbers to the right of the decimal point represent whole numbers, and numbers to the left of the decimal point represent quantities less than one. *Numbers to the left of the decimal point represent whole numbers, and numbers to the right of the decimal point represent quantities less than one.*

2. True. With respect to rounding, pharmacy numbers must be measurable and practical.

3. True. Percentages also convert simply to decimals. Just remove the % sign, and move the decimal point two places to the left.

4. True. The symbol μ has been used as an abbreviation for micro, but this is an unsafe symbol because it can be confused with an "m."

5. False. The avoirdupois system is a Spanish system of mass that includes grams and liters. *This is a French system that includes ounces and pounds.*

6. False. Ideal body weight (IBW) is an estimate of how much a patient should weigh, based on his or her height and gender and is expressed as pounds. *IBW is expressed as kg.*

7. False. Body mass index (BMI) is a measure of body fat based on height and weight and is commonly used in medication calculations. *The BMI is generally not used in medication calculations, but it may be mentioned in the pharmacy and in the literature.*

8. True. Specific gravity is the ratio of the weight of the compound to the weight of the same amount of water.

9. False. Specific gravity is expressed in grams. *Generally, units do not appear with specific gravity.*

10. True. In pharmacy calculations, specific gravity and density are used interchangeably.

11. True. When calculating concentration percentages of medications, if the product does not contain active ingredient, its concentration is 0%; if the product is pure active ingredient, its concentration is 100%.

12. False. Some pharmacy mixtures are created by adding two solids together. When this occurs, the percentage strength is measured in weight in weight (w/w) or grams of drug/10 grams of mixture. *The percentage strength is measured in weight in weight (w/w) or grams of drug/100 grams of mixture.*

Fill in the Blank Key

1. X

2. L

3. C

4. V

5. M

6. ss

7. Numerator, denominator

8. Ratio

9. Alligation

10. Apothecary

Short Answer Key

1. When presented with a Roman numeral, it is important to pay attention to the order of the symbols. First, identify the largest Roman numeral. If more than one numeral of the same quantity is present, then add them together. Second, locate the smaller numerals. If the smaller numerals are to the right of the largest numeral(s), the quantity of the small numerals is added to the largest numeral. If the smaller numerals are to the left of the largest numeral(s), the quantity of the smaller numerals is subtracted from the largest numeral(s).

2. When adding fractions, there are three simple steps to remember:

   a. Make sure all the fractions have common denominators. The easiest way to do this is to enlarge the fraction by either multiplying both parts of the fraction by the denominator of the other or by using the lowest (or least) common denominator.

   b. Add the numerators.

   c. Reduce to the simplest fraction or mixed number.

3. When multiplying fractions, it is not necessary to convert to common denominators. Steps to multiply fractions:

   a. Multiply the numerators.

   b. Multiply the denominators.

   c. Express your answer as a fraction.

   d. Simplify the fraction.

4. When dividing fractions, it is not necessary to convert to common denominators. Steps to divide fractions:

   a. Convert the second fraction (divisor) to its reciprocal; that is, trade the places of the numerator and the denominator.

   b. Multiply the first fraction by the second fraction's reciprocal.

   c. Simplify the fraction.

5. Body mass index (BMI) is a measure of body fat based on height and weight. This value is used to determine if a patient is underweight, of normal weight, overweight, or obese. The BMI is not generally used in medication calculations, but it may be mentioned in the pharmacy and in the literature.

   Ideal body weight (IBW) is an estimate of how much a patient should weigh, based on his or her height and gender. IBW is expressed as kg.

   Body surface area (BSA) is a value that takes the patient's weight and height into account and is expressed as m2. BSA values are frequently used to calculate doses of chemotherapeutic agents. Several similar equations are used such as the Mosteller formula.

Crossword Puzzle Key

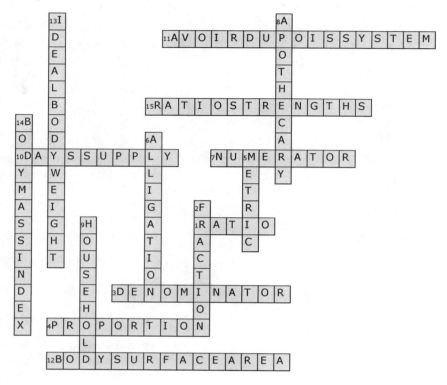

Chapter 15 Answer Keys

Multiple Choice Key

1. d. All of the above.

2. d. All of the above.

3. c. All of the above.

4. a. The medication is aqueous (water-based) or nonaqueous.

5. a. Allow another individual to reproduce the same formulation at a later date.

6. d. All of the above.

7. c. To use the smallest graduate that will hold the volume to be measured.

8. a. The mortar is the "bowl" and the pestle is the "stirrer."

9. c. Compatibility in the final preparation is considered in the selection.

10. d. Reduce particle size in preparations.

Matching Key

1. L. A compounding method of incorporating a solid (i.e., powder) into an ointment. A small amount of a levigating agent is added to the powder to form a paste, which is then incorporated into the ointment.

2. D. A date that is given to a medication noting when it should no longer be used; also referred to as the expiration date.

3. P. A medication individualized for a specific patient that requires the mixing of ingredients in a pharmacy and is based on a prescription or drug order.

4. T. A non-reusable container designed to hold a quantity of drug to be administered as a single dose.

5. K. An ingredient that is necessary to prepare the formulation, but is not intended to cause a pharmacologic response. Inactive ingredients may also be referred to as inert ingredients, added ingredients or substances, or excipients, and include, for example, colorants, flavorants, sweeteners, and wetting agents.

6. J. Compounding equipment used to measure the volume of liquid ingredients; generally glass or plastic cylinders and conicals.

7. I. Compounding technique used to ensure the uniform mixing when there is a wide discrepancy in amounts of individual ingredients. The preparer starts with the smallest ingredient amount and mixes it with an equal amount (estimated by sight) of the next smallest ingredient amount and continues adding and doubling the size until all ingredients are integrated.

8. N. Compounds prepared in a pharmacy that do not require strict aseptic technique and include preparations such as oral and topical medications.

9. R. Compounds prepared in a pharmacy using strict aseptic technique, including preparations such as injections, ophthalmic solutions, and irrigation solutions.

10. Q. Defined in USP-NF as the extent to which a preparation retains, within specified limits and throughout its period of storage and use, the same properties and characteristics that it possessed at the time of compounding.

11. G. Includes the facilities (i.e., compounding area) and equipment in the pharmacy.

12. A. Ingredient in the compounded preparation that is responsible for the therapeutic or pharmaceutical action of the medication.

13. E. Often called "bubble packs." Composed of a plastic bubble that forms a cavity for the medication. The package is then sealed with a backing material that also acts as a label.

14. U. Pumps that allow the user to preset a volume to be dispensed into a container on the basis of the draw back setting.

15. O. Pumps with a series of roller wheels that press against tubing to force a volume of liquid down the length of the tubing.

16. H. Repackaging quantities of medications that will be used within a short period of time.

17. S. The act of mixing powders or crushing tablets using a mortar and pestle (i.e., solid is rubbed with mortar and pestle) until a state of fine, evenly sized particles is achieved.

18. B. The compounding record for a batch, usually filed by lot number.

19. C. The periodic repackaging of large quantities of medications in unit-dose or single-unit packages.

20. M. Typically occurs in licensed manufacturing facilities and includes the production, conversion, and/or processing of a drug, generally in bulk quantities and without a prescription or medication order.

21. F. Usually takes place in a pharmacy and includes the preparation, mixing, packaging, and labeling of a small quantity of a drug based on a practitioner's prescription or medication order for a specific patient.

True or False Key

1. False. When pharmacies compound both sterile and nonsterile preparations, the compounding area for sterile preparations is also used for compounding nonsterile preparations. *In these pharmacies, the compounding area for sterile preparations is separate and distinct from the area used for compounding nonsterile preparations.*

2. False. If a patient needs a drug that has been withdrawn from the market by the FDA, the patient should ask a compounding pharmacy to order the ingredients and compound the medication. *Any drug that is withdrawn from the market by the FDA should not be used.*

3. True. Preparations should contain at least 90%, but not more than 110%, of the labeled active ingredient, unless more restrictive guidelines apply.

4. False. To be as efficient as possible, several similar preparations may be compounded at one time in the compounding area if the compounding personnel are experienced. *Only one preparation should be compounded at one time in the compounding area to avoid errors and cross-contamination.*

5. False. Patient counseling is not required for compounded medications. *Patient counseling is important with all medications, including compounded formulations. The patient should be counseled by the pharmacist on the correct use, storage, beyond-use date, and evidence of instability in the compounded medication.*

6. False. Because they do not cause pharmacologic activity, inactive ingredients are not a necessary part of the product, and the specific chemicals used as excipients do not need to be named in the formula. *Inactive ingredients are a necessary part of the product, and the specific chemicals used as excipients must be named in the formula.*

7. False. Once a class A torsion balance is calibrated, it does not need to be recalibrated as long as it remains on a stable and solid surface. *The balance must be maintained and calibrated regularly.*

8. False. The bottom of the meniscus should be read at counter level. *The bottom of the meniscus should be read at eye level.*

9. False. Wedgewood mortars are preferable when mixing liquids or preparing solutions, suspensions, or lotions, adding flavoring oils and coloring. *It is preferable to use glass mortars when mixing liquids, preparing solutions, suspensions, or lotions as well as when adding flavoring oils and coloring.*

10. True. An ointment slab or ointment paper may be used for preparing and mixing creams and ointments.

11. False. Numerous capsule sizes and colors are available for human and veterinary use. Sizes of capsules for humans range from No. 000 to No. 5. No. 000 is the smallest, and No. 5 is the largest. *No. 000 is the largest, and No. 5 is the smallest.*

12. True. Extemporaneous repackaging is also known as "just-in-time" packaging.

13. False. End-product testing is performed for all repackaging processes. *End-product testing is not generally performed for basic repackaging processes.*

14. False. Peristaltic pumps need less recalibrating than volumetric pumps and are more accurate and reliable for delivering fluid volumes of less than 10 mL. *Volumetric pumps need less recalibrating than peristaltic pumps and are more accurate and reliable for delivering fluid volumes of less than 10 mL.*

Fill in the Blank Key

1. 795
2. Stability
3. Beyond-use
4. Master formula
5. Meniscus
6. Trituration
7. Levigation
8. Geometric dilution
9. National Drug Code
10. Extemporaneous
11. Batch
12. Checkpoints

Short Answer Key

1. Prior to the technician compounding the preparation, the pharmacist clinically evaluates the appropriateness of the prescription or drug order in terms of safety and intended use for the patient. In addition, as these steps are reviewed, it is important to understand that only one preparation should be compounded at one time in the compounding area to avoid errors and cross-contamination.

    a. Calculate the amount of ingredients needed for the preparation.

    b. Identify equipment needed to compound the preparation.

    c. Wash hands and wear proper attire.

    d. Clean the compounding area and needed equipment.

    e. Collect all materials and ingredients needed.

    f. Compound the preparation following a formulation record (file of individually compounded preparations) or prescription and according to the art and science of pharmacy.

    g. Document name on the compounding record/log.

    h. Label the final preparation appropriately.

    i. Properly clean and store all equipment.

2. Mortars and pestles are used to crush, grind, and blend various medicinal ingredients. Trituration is achieved by moving the pestle in a circular motion in the mortar. Mortars are available in a variety of materials such as glass, porcelain, and Wedgewood. Glass mortars are preferable when mixing liquids or preparing solutions, suspensions, or lotions. Glass mortars are also non-staining and, therefore, should be used when adding flavoring oils and coloring. Wedgewood mortars have a rough interior surface and are ideal for intense grinding and trituration to reduce particle size. Wedgewood mortars stain easily and are porous; therefore, extra care must be taken when cleaning Wedgewood to ensure that all particles are removed to avoid cross contamination. Porcelain mortars are also very durable and are often used for blending powders and reducing particle size. Porcelain mortars have a glazed interior surface that is less porous than Wedgewood.

3. Each step of the compounding process should be documented. USP Chapter 795 requires pharmacies to maintain a formulation record, also known as the master formula, and a compounding record for each compounded preparation. The formulation record is an individual

record (like a recipe) that is stored in a file with other formulas. They are usually filed alphabetically, so it is easy to find the desired formula. This record includes a listing of the ingredients, compounding equipment, and instructions for preparing the formula. The goal of documentation is for quality purposes, to allow another individual to reproduce the same formulation at a later date, and to trace each ingredient in the compound, if necessary. The compounding record is the log (or record) of an actual compounded preparation (i.e., based on an individual prescription or drug order) or batch being prepared (i.e., for compounds prepared in anticipation of orders). It includes manufacturer and lot numbers of chemicals used, the date of preparation, an internal identification number (commonly called a lot number), a beyond-use date, the names of the individuals who prepared and verified the preparation, and any other pertinent information regarding the preparation. The compounding record for a batch (batch record) is usually filed by lot number, whereas the compounding record for an individual prescription or drug order is a chronological list of preparations made. Depending upon state laws and regulations, the formulation and compounding records may be maintained as paper copies or electronic files in the pharmacy.

4. Labeling is the responsibility of the dispenser who should take into account the nature of the drug repackaged, the characteristics of the containers, and the storage conditions to which the medication may be subjected in order to determine a beyond-use date for the label. USP offers standards for determining an appropriate expiration date in the absence of published stability data, "For nonsterile solid and liquid dosage forms that are packaged in single-unit and unit-dose containers, the beyond use date shall be 1 year from the date packaged or the expiration date on the manufacturer's container, whichever is earlier." Considerable technical advances have occurred in the area of labeling, partly as a result of using computers in institutional practice. In particular, personal computers have greatly improved the quality and efficiency of the label production process.

Current federal labeling requirements are described in the ASHP Technical Assistance Bulletin on Single Unit and Unit Dose Packages of Drugs. The technical bulletin states that the nonproprietary name (generic name), proprietary name (brand name) if appropriate, dosage form, strength, amount delivered in package, notes (such as storage conditions, preparation, or administration instructions), expiration date, and control number or lot number should appear on the package. Inclusion of a barcode on repackaged items is highly recommended and is necessary to facilitate bedside barcode scanning in hospitals. Most computerized packaging machines include the ability to include a bar code to identify the medication in the package. Some labels are applied manually to the finished product. Newer semi-automated and automated repackaging machines have printers built in so the label can be printed on the package prior to the dosage form being inserted.

Word Search Key

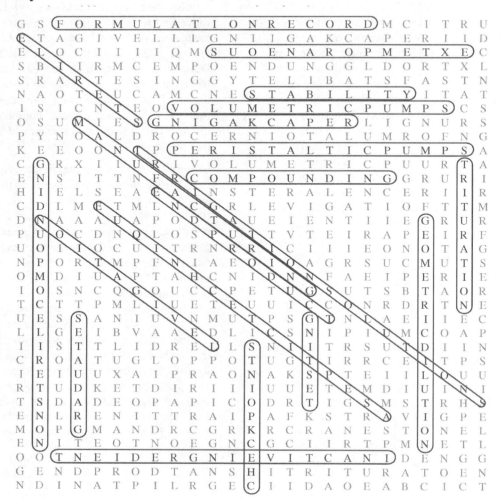

Chapter 16 Answer Keys

Multiple Choice Key

1. d. All of the above.

2. d. All of the above.

3. d. All of the above.

4. d. All of the above.

5. b. 10 units/mL or 100 units/mL.

6. a. High efficiency particulate air or HEPA filter.

7. b. 6 inches.

8. c. 15-30.

9. b. 70%.

10. d. Up-and-down direction, starting at the HEPA and working toward the outer edge of the hood.

Matching Key

1. A. Dextrose

2. D. Amino acids

3. B. Sodium chloride

4. B. Potassium chloride

5. B. Potassium phosphate

6. B. Calcium gluconate

7. B. Magnesium sulfate

8. E. MVI

9. C. 10% fat emulsion

10. E. Vitamin K

True or False Key

1. True. IVs may be administered to patients at home by their families rather than by nurses.

2. True. When drugs are injected directly into the body, the body's barriers to infection are bypassed.

3. True. Drug incompatibilities may involve other drugs, containers, or solutions.

4. False. Extravasation is a very minor problem, seldom causing any complications. *Extravasation and infiltration can be painful and usually require that the IV be restarted in a different location, and some drugs such as certain chemotherapy agents may cause severe tissue damage if they infiltrate the tissue. While there are medications to alleviate some of the effects of the drug and hot and cold compresses to arrest progression, in some cases the tissue damage can be so severe that it requires surgery or even loss of the limb.*

5. False. When an IV solution is sterilized, pyrogens are removed. *A pyrogen can be present even after a solution has been sterilized.*

6. False. When drugs are added to the IV solution to prepare the final sterile product, the drug is referred to as the admixture and the final product is referred to as the additive. *When drugs are added to the IV solution to prepare the final sterile product, the drug is referred to as the additive and the final product is referred to as the admixture.*

7. False. All laminar flow workbenches should be cleaned with alcohol. *Plexiglas sides, found on some types of laminar flow workbenches, should be cleaned with warm, soapy water rather than alcohol because the alcohol will dry out the Plexiglas and cause it to become cloudy and possibly cracked.*

8. True. Nothing should be permitted to come in contact with the HEPA filter.

9. False. Only those objects essential to product preparation should be placed in the LAFW such as pens and labels. *Only those objects essential to product preparation should be placed in the LAFW. Do not put paper, pens, labels, or trays into the hood.*

10. False. Jewelry may be worn on the hands or wrists when working in the LAFW as long as appropriate clean room attire covers all exposures. *Jewelry should not be worn on the hands or wrists when working in the LAFW since it may introduce bacteria or particles into the clean work area or compromise the glove barrier.*

11. True. Every entry into a sterile product area should include scrubbing your hands, nails, wrists, and forearms to elbows thoroughly for at least 30 seconds with a brush, warm water, and appropriate bactericidal soap before performing aseptic manipulations.

12. True. Due to their toxicity, solutions with preservatives should not be used for epidural or intrathecal dosage forms and should only be used with caution in pediatric or neonatal preparations.

13. False. To withdraw the solution from an ampule, a needle with a 5-micron filter in the hub should be used for withdrawing contents and expelling contents. *To withdraw the solution, either use a filter needle and change to a regular needle before expelling the contents, or start with a regular needle and change to a filter needle before expelling the contents. Either way, the filter needle must not be used for both withdrawing from the ampule or expelling from the syringe because doing so would nullify the filtering effect. Usually, the medication is withdrawn from the ampule with a regular needle, and then the needle is changed to a filter needle before pushing the drug out of the syringe.*

14. True. All hazardous drugs should be identified by distinctive labels, indicating that the product requires special handling.

15. True. Precipitation may occur if the wrong sequence or concentrations of electrolytes are added to an IV bag.

Fill in the Blank Key

1. Peripherally inserted central catheter (PICC) or PICC line

2. Extravasation

3. Pyrogens

4. Phlebitis

5. 100

6. Piggyback

7. Add-Vantage®

8. Smart pump

9. Elastomeric infusion device (EID)

10. Aseptic

11. 5

12. Vertical

13. Ampules

14. 797

Short Answer Key

1. Infection—Infections can result if a product contaminated with microorganisms or pathogens is infused into a patient. Human touch contamination (improper product handling) continues to be the most common source of IV-related contamination.

Air embolus is caused if air is infused into the patient from the IV line. In adults, it takes 15 to 20 mL of air given quickly to result in harm. Infants and pediatric patients are adversely affected by much lower amounts of air. Air-eliminating filters are available on some IV sets, which also stop air bubbles and add another measure of safety.

Bleeding may be caused by intravenous therapy. When the IV catheter is removed, bleeding may occur around the catheter site. Also, if the patient has a condition that results in prolonged bleeding time or is receiving an anticoagulant medication, extra care and caution should be used, especially when removing the catheter.

When a patient has an allergic reaction to a substance given parenterally, the reaction is usually more severe than if the same substance was given by another route because substances given parenterally cannot be retrieved like substances given by other routes. When a drug that has caused allergic reactions in a large number of patients is given intravenously, the patient should be monitored closely. If the likelihood of an allergic reaction is especially high, a test dose (a small amount of the drug) often referred to as a challenge, may be given to see how the patient reacts before administering the full dose of the medication if there is no alternative therapy allowing for risk mitigation.

Some drugs are incompatible with other drugs, containers, or solutions. If an incompatibility exists, the drug may precipitate, be inactivated, or adhere to the container. These outcomes are undesirable and may be difficult to detect with the naked eye. A visual inspection of the final product should always be performed to observe any cloudiness, coring, or signs of irregularity. Solutions with known or detectable incompatibilities should not be administered to patients.

Extravasation occurs when the IV catheter punctures and exits the vein under the skin, causing drugs to infuse or infiltrate into the tissue. Extravasation may happen when the catheter is being inserted or after it is in place, if the extremity with the IV catheter is moved or flexed too much. Using a stiff arm board to prevent excessive movement near the catheter site may help maintain regular flow and prevent extravasation and infiltration. Extravasation and infiltration can be painful and usually requires that the IV be restarted in a different location. Some drugs such as certain chemotherapy agents may cause severe tissue damage if they infiltrate the tissue. While there are medications to alleviate some of the effects of the drug and hot and cold compresses to arrest progression, in some cases the tissue damage can be so severe that it requires surgery or even loss of the limb.

Particulate matter refers to unwanted particles present in parenteral products. Particulate matter that is injected into the bloodstream can cause adverse effects to the patient. Some examples of particulate matter are microscopic glass fragments, hair, lint or cotton fibers, cardboard fragments, undissolved drug particles, and fragments of rubber stoppers, known as cores. Improvements in manufacturing processes have greatly reduced the presence of particulates in commercially available products. Similar care must be taken in the pharmacy so that particulate matter is not introduced into products. When using glass ampules, for example, inline filters are required to prevent glass fragments from entering the compounded sterile product. All products should be visually inspected for particulate matter before dispensing. Some institutions may additionally use inline filters to help minimize the amount of particulate that reaches the patient, especially in situations where medications need to be prepared in emergency situations outside the controlled environment of a pharmacy.

Pyrogens, the by-products or remnants of bacteria, can cause reactions (e.g., fever and chills) if injected in large enough amounts. Since a pyrogen can be present even after a solution has been sterilized, great care must be taken to ensure that these substances are not present in quantities that would harm the patient via filtration when appropriate. If the pyrogen is smaller than the filter being used; however, it may be introduced into the bloodstream.

Phlebitis—Phlebitis, or irritation of the vein, may be caused by the IV catheter, the drug being administered (due to its chemical properties or its concentration), the location of the IV site, a fast rate of administration, or the presence of particulate matter. The patient usually feels pain or discomfort along the path of the vein, which is often severe. Red streaking may also occur. If phlebitis is caused by a particular drug, it may be helpful to further dilute the drug, give it more slowly, or give it via an IV catheter placed in a larger vein with a higher, faster moving volume of blood.

2. Compounding area counters, easily cleanable work surfaces, and floors should be cleaned daily, while walls, ceilings, and storage shelving should be cleaned monthly at a minimum. Segregated compounding areas must be separate from normal pharmacy operations, nonessential equipment, and other materials that produce particles. For example, the introduction of cardboard into the clean room environment should be avoided. Traffic flow into the sterile compounding area should be minimized. Trash should be removed frequently and regularly. Care should be taken to take the trash cans outside of the IV room before pulling the trash or otherwise removing it from the container.

3. There are two common types of laminar flow workbenches, horizontal flow and vertical flow. *Horizontal LAFW.* LAFWs that sweep filtered air from the back of the hood to the front are called horizontal LAFWs. Horizontal flow workbenches use an electrical blower to draw contaminated room air through a prefilter. The prefilter, which is similar to a furnace filter, only removes gross contaminants and should be cleaned or replaced on a regular basis. The prefiltered air is then pressurized in a plenum to ensure that a consistent distribution of airflow is presented to the final filtering apparatus. The final filter constitutes the entire back portion of the hood's work area. This high efficiency particulate air, or HEPA filter, removes 99.97% of particles that are 0.3 micron or larger, thereby eliminating airborne microorganisms, which are usually 0.5 microns or larger.

Vertical LAFW. Laminar flow workbenches with a vertical flow of filtered air are also available. In vertical LAFWs, HEPA filtered air emerges from the top and passes downward through the work area. Because exposure to antineoplastic (anticancer) drugs may be harmful, they should only be prepared in vertical LAFWs so that the risk of exposure to airborne drug particulates is minimized. The types of vertical LAFW used for the preparation of antineoplastics confine airflow within the hood and are referred to as biological safety cabinets (BSCs). If possible, prepare sterile hazardous drugs in a Class II BSC. The front air barrier of the BSC protects the handler from contact with hazardous drug dusts and aerosols that are generated in the work zone. Room air is pulled into the front intake grill and filtered through a HEPA filter. The air then passes vertically or downward,

through the work zone. The air that has passed through the work zone goes through front intake and rear exhaust grilles, passes through a separate HEPA filter, and is recirculated through the work zone or exhausted to the outside. Placing objects on or near the front intake or rear exhaust grilles may obstruct the airflow and reduce the effectiveness of the cabinet.

There are several types of Class II BSCs. Type A BSCs pump about 30% of the air out the hood exhaust after it passes through a HEPA filter. This air is then circulated to the room or exhausted to the outside, depending on how the hood is vented. Type B BSCs send air from the work zone through a HEPA filter and then to the outside of the building through an auxiliary exhaust system. Type B BSCs offer greater protection because filtered air is sent outside the building, and they have a faster inward flow of air. It is preferable to have the BSC exhausted directly to the outside through dedicated venting rather than venting into the general hospital circulation.

4. In some institutions, it is the responsibility of the pharmacy to prime the line with the chemotherapeutic agent. Additional precautions will need to be taken if this is the case. To properly prime the line, obtain the proper IV tubing and the IV bag being prepared. Then unwrap the tubing inside the BSC. Close the tubing flow by using the roller clamp, remove the tubing tip, and place it aside. Insert the tubing spike (located above the fluid chamber) into the IV bag and slowly roll open the roller clamp, allowing IV fluid to flow through the tubing. Follow the fluid until the IV fluid reaches the end of the tubing. Allow a few drops of fluid to exit the tubing and then close the roller clamp as well as the on/off clamp and replace the tubing tip. Proper priming should have minimal to no air bubbles in the tubing. Proper manipulation of the roller clamp will ensure minimal bubbles. Priming the IV tubing should be done prior to preparing any chemotherapy IV bags.

5. Spill kits are used for the spill of hazardous drugs and contain protective gear, eye protection, a respirator, utility and latex gloves, a disposable gown or coveralls, and shoe covers. They also contain the equipment needed to clean up the spill: a disposable scoop, a puncture- and leak-resistant plastic container for disposing of glass fragments, absorbent spill pads, gauze and disposable toweling, absorbent powder, and sealable, thick plastic waste disposal bags.

Crossword Puzzle Key

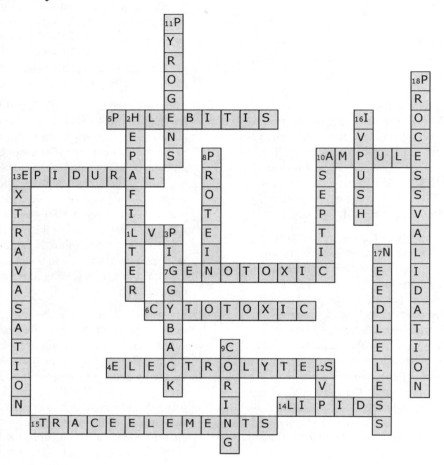

Chapter 17 Answer Keys

Multiple Choice Key

1. a. The different monitoring, measuring, and reporting techniques used.

2. c. 19%.

3. c. Performance lapses or failure to follow established procedures.

4. d. At any point during the medication use process.

5. c. Helps to classify errors, but some errors may fit in several of the categories.

6. e. All of the above.

7. d. Forgetting to administer the ADD-Vantage® IV admixture bag.

8. e. All of the above.

9. d. Prescribing error.

10. c. 19.

Matching Key

You will see that there are sometimes several answers that could be correct, which emphasizes the chapter's point that classifying and counting errors depends on what the institution's policy is. For instance, if one error causes another error, is that counted as two errors or do you count it as the first error? There is no perfect system, but the current system is a great start.

1. K. Mrs. Jones took her antibiotic for 6 days until she felt better, although she was supposed to take the medication for 10 days.

2. D. George was having stomach problems so his neigh-

bor shared his PPI medication because it worked so well for him.

3. L. At St. Francis Hospital, all medications must be given within 1 hour of the assigned administration time. Nurse Cratchet gave Bob his 0900 medication at 0800.

4. E. Fred was supposed to get 13 units of insulin for a blood glucose reading of 160-170. His BG was 169. He received 12 units of insulin.

5. G. Greta was mixing up a bottle of Cleocin Pediatric. She was supposed to add 75 mL of water to make a total of 100 mL of solution. She only added 60 mL of water, so she changed the total quantity to 80 mL and changed the directions to make sure the patient got the correct dose.

6. B or K. Justine forgot to take her vitamin D on Tuesday.

7. J. Nurse Annie was supposed to give Frank 100 mg of atenolol each day as long as his blood pressure was greater than 160/100. His blood pressure has been over 160/100 every day for 3 weeks, so she skipped taking the blood pressure reading today and gave him his medication anyway.

8. A. The physician prescribed ciprofloxacin for a 7-year-old child. The pharmacist called the physician and reminded him that this class of drugs should be avoided in children.

9. A causing H. The physician's directions were for Boric Acid Capsules 500 mg q day. The nurse gave the patient this dose by mouth. The intended route was vaginal.

10. L. The expiration date on the bottle of naproxen 500 mg was 7-10. The patient received a prescription of naproxen 500 g #20 1 tab bid on 7-3-10. *An expiration date of 7-10 means until the end of the month or 7-31-10.*

True or False Key

1. False. Some of the errors as defined in the ASHP guidelines apply primarily to patients in health care facilities and do not apply to other settings such as home health care, clinic, and physician office settings or outpatient pharmacy practice settings. *Actually, these same definitions can be applied to home health care, clinic, and physician office settings as well as the outpatient pharmacy practice settings.*

2. False. There have been numerous and thorough studies of medication errors in hospitals. *Few studies provide a complete and thorough evaluation of errors within the entire medication use process.*

3. False. Errors occurring earlier in the medication use process (in the prescribing phase) are less likely to be detected and corrected than those occurring later in the process (in administration). *It has been observed that errors occurring earlier in the medication use process (in the prescribing phase) are more likely to be detected and corrected than those occurring later in the process (in administration).*

4. True. A good general rule to follow is to question any dose that requires less than ½ or more than 2 of the dosage unit (tablet, capsule, teaspoonful).

5. False. The recipient of a verbal or telephone order should immediately repeat the order to the prescriber and then immediately write down the order to ensure clarity. *The recipient of a verbal or telephone order should immediately write down the order and read it back to the prescriber to ensure clarity.*

6. True. The pharmacist should clarify ambiguous doses before the technician processes the order.

7. True. Read the label at least three times to help prevent medication errors: when you remove it from the shelf, as it is being prepared, and as the finished product is set aside for the pharmacist to check.

8. False. The abbreviation "qid" is considered unsafe by the Joint Commission. *QD and qod are considered unsafe, but qid is not.*

9. False. The correct way to write Coumadin ½ mg using decimals is "Coumadin .5 mg." *The correct way to write Coumadin ½ mg using decimals is "Coumadin 0.5 mg."*

10. False. The correct way to abbreviate microgram is µg. *The correct way to abbreviate microgram is mcg.*

Fill in the Blank Key

1. Misadventure
2. Prescribing
3. Omission
4. Wrong time
5. Unauthorized drug
6. Improper dose
7. Wrong dosage form
8. Wrong drug preparation
9. Wrong administration technique
10. Deteriorated drug
11. Monitoring
12. Compliance

Short Answer Key

1. Factors within the workplace can contribute to medication errors. Inadequate lighting, poorly designed work spaces, and inefficient workflow can make it difficult to perform assigned duties accurately. Cluttered work spaces and stock areas can increase the risk of picking up the wrong drug. The many distractions and interruptions, including phone calls, in a busy pharmacy can cause loss of concentration. Many modern pharmacies rely on specialized equipment and computers to assist in filling prescriptions. Improper maintenance of this equipment can result in unacceptable performance or may necessitate the use of older, unfamiliar, or cumbersome manual systems when the equipment breaks down. For example, failure to properly maintain a balance can result in an inaccurate measure of medication components for a compounded prescription and ultimately a wrong dose error. Routine maintenance schedules should be followed to prevent equipment malfunction. Technicians should be trained on the use and maintenance of such equipment. Operating manuals should be available in the pharmacy for troubleshooting when a problem occurs. Scheduling of staff members and the frequency of rotating shifts have been shown to correlate with error rates. Other factors, such as staffing levels and amount of supervision, are also work environment issues to consider.

   The frequency with which drug products are changed because of changes in purchasing contracts may lead to unfamiliarity with products among the staff. Significant changes should be communicated to the staff, and product labels should be read carefully. Untrained, inadequately trained, or inexperienced personnel may be unfamiliar with drug names, doses, or uses of agents, which limits their ability to recognize inappropriate orders and circumstances. New technological advances make keeping up with drug use difficult even for experienced health care practitioners. The important thing is for technicians to recognize their limits and work within them, just as nurses, pharmacists, and physicians are trained to do.

   Relying on memory instead of checking references (e.g., dilution charts, maximum dosage ranges) or performing complicated calculations without a double check stage can result in errors. It is a technician's responsibility to help prevent medication errors by questioning unusual or unfamiliar orders. When abnormal or unfamiliar situations arise, it is always best to consult references and others before making a decision or taking action. Being aware of a potential error and not knowing what to do about it, thinking that someone else will catch it, or feeling intimidated by a pharmacist or supervisor increases the chances that an actual error will take place. The lack of knowledge of medication errors and how to avoid them also contributes to medication errors. Not being familiar with common errors or medications most frequently involved in errors might cause one to think that medication errors are infrequent. The medication errors most frequently reported to the USP in 2002 involved albuterol, insulin, morphine, potassium chloride, heparin, and warfarin. Of these six medications, all but albuterol were most frequently involved in errors that were associated with patient harm or death.

2. Sometimes the systems that people work within present numerous opportunities for errors. Failure mode and effects analysis (FMEA), also called failure mode effect and criticality analysis (FMECA), is a systematic evaluation of a process or system used to predict the opportunity for and severity of errors at various steps in the process. FMEA focuses on finding flaws within a system that create opportunities for individuals to make errors. It evaluates the "how" and "why" of an error instead of the "who." The first step in evaluating a system or process using FMEA is to describe in detail the individual steps involved in the overall process from start to finish. Use of a flow diagram is helpful to create a visual representation of the process. The next step is to list the potential opportunities for failure at each stage. Then, the effects of these failures on the process and their root causes are described. The severity, likelihood of occurrence, and probability of actually identifying the failure are then estimated. The criticality index is determined by multiplying these three estimates. Steps that have the highest criticality index should be addressed first because improvements in these areas have the greatest potential for reducing the risk for error. After making changes to the process, FMEA should be performed again to determine the effectiveness of these changes. An acute care hospital in California used the FMEA system to reduce IV pump-related medication errors. One year after implementation of several error reduction strategies identified during the FMEA, pump-related medication errors had decreased significantly.

3. *Once an error has occurred,* it is important to thoroughly examine the error to learn why it occurred and how such an error can be avoided in the future. A root cause analysis (RCA) is a process that examines the contributing factors regarding why and how an error (or near miss) occurred. There are usually several factors that led to the error. A root cause analysis consists of five steps:

a. Establish a team of appropriate personnel to conduct the root cause analysis. This team may include pharmacists, technicians, nurses, prescribers, risk management representatives, or other allied health personnel. The team should seek management support and establish meeting times and locations.

b. Describe the event in detail. As much information as possible about the event should be obtained, and the people directly involved in the event should be interviewed. The description of the event is then revised to include any new findings.

c. Diagram the steps that led up to the error to help determine the root cause. The steps should be described in chronological order and thoroughly examined for inconsistencies or weaknesses. Based on this information, propose a summary of causes.

d. Develop a specific action plan to address the identified causes of the error. Some of the action plans might be implemented immediately, whereas others may be more long term.

e. Develop outcome measures in order to determine if the action plan is effective. The outcome measures should evaluate whether the actions taken actually prevent similar errors.

4. Reports show that numerous medication errors are caused by errors in mathematical calculations. Miscalculation of doses can lead to serious patient harm or even death. Calculation errors are made by prescribers, pharmacists checking doses for appropriateness or calculating doses, technicians compounding products, and nurses preparing or administering doses. Even with the use of calculators and computers, health care personnel frequently make calculation errors. The pediatric population is particularly at risk for calculation errors. It is not uncommon for pediatric doses to be determined by the patient's weight, requiring an interim step to calculate the final dose. Many drugs are not available in pediatric formulations, so adult formulations must be diluted or manipulated multiple times to get the appropriate dose. Personnel with many years of experience are just as likely to make mathematical errors as inexperienced personnel.

Calculation errors are often made by using the wrong concentration of stock solutions, misplacing a decimal point, or using wrong conversions. Personnel also neglect to double-check their work, or rely on their memory instead of looking up a conversion. In some cases, they fail to ask themselves, "Does the answer seem reasonable?" Another way to decrease the risk of a calculation error is to ask a pharmacist or another technician to double check the calculation prior to preparing the product. The calculation should be performed independently and should be compared with the original answer. This system is an effective way to prevent calculation errors.

Misplacing a decimal point by one place results in errors tenfold greater than or less than intended. For drugs with a narrow therapeutic range (e.g., digoxin, phenytoin, warfarin, gentamicin), the consequences can be significant. Decimal point errors can occur as a result of a miscalculation, and also when writing orders or instructions. Failure to write a leading zero in front of a number less than one (e.g., .1 mg instead of 0.1 mg) can result in the number being read as a whole number (1 mg). Writing unnecessary trailing zeros can also be confusing (e.g., 10.0 mg instead of 10 mg, which could be misinterpreted as 100 mg). Medication order sheets with lines can sometimes cause a decimal point to be overlooked on the copy that is sent to the pharmacy. Medication orders that are received via fax should be reviewed carefully since artifact (insignificant markings on the page) might cause the order to be misinterpreted. When writing numbers, a leading zero should always be used with a decimal point for numbers less than one (0.1 mg, not .1 mg), and a decimal point and trailing zero should never be used for whole numbers (10 mg, not 10.0 mg). Technicians must be aware of the potential for decimal point errors due to misplaced or missing decimal points when interpreting orders, and questionable orders should be brought to the attention of the pharmacist.

Word Search Key

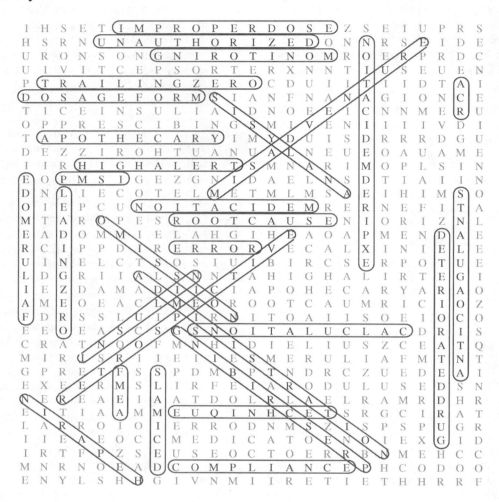

Chapter 18 Answer Keys

Multiple Choice Key

1. c. Durable medical equipment.

2. c. 70-130 mg/dL.

3. d. All of the above.

4. d. All of the above.

5. a. The abdomen.

6. d. All of the above.

7. d. All of the above.

8. b. Diabetic ketoacidosis (DKA).

9. b. 60-100 beats per minute.

10. d. All of the above.

Matching I Key

1. D. Insulin detemir (Levemir)

2. A. Insulin lispro (Humalog)

3. B. Regular Human (Humulin R, Novolin R)

4. A. Insulin glulisine (Apidra)

5. A. Insulin aspart (Novolog)

6. C. NPH (Humulin N, Novolin N)

7. D. Insulin glargine (Lantus)

Matching II Key

1. B. Absorbent bed pads
2. A. Blood glucose meters
3. B. Blood glucose test strips and lancets
4. A. Blood pressure monitors
5. A. Braces
6. A. Canes
7. A. Commode and shower chairs
8. A. Crutches
9. B. Diapers
10. B. Dressing materials (bandages, gauze dressings, tape)
11. B. Exam gloves
12. A. Home oxygen equipment
13. A. Hospital beds
14. A. Infusion pumps
15. B. Insulin syringes and pen needles
16. A. Nebulizers
17. B. Ostomy supplies
18. A. Scooters
19. A. Suction pumps
20. A. Walkers
21. A. Wheelchairs

True or False Key

1. False. Any pharmacy that obtains the correct Medicare Part B Forms may bill Medicare for medical equipment. *The Centers for Medicare and Medicaid Services require that all suppliers of durable medical equipment, prosthetics, orthotics, and supplies be accredited to bill Medicare Part B. As of January 1, 2010, pharmacies that supply this type of equipment must be Medicare accredited.*

2. False. Hyperglycemia (high blood glucose) and hypoglycemia (low blood glucose) can be identified with the use of insulin pens. *Hyperglycemia (high blood glucose) and hypoglycemia (low blood glucose) can be identified with the use blood glucose meters.*

3. True. Insulin is classified according to its action (rapid-acting, short-acting, intermediate acting, or long-acting).

4. False. The advantage of durable insulin pens is that they are disposable. *Durable insulin pens are reusable.*

5. False. Most disposable insulin pens contain 3 mL or 3000 units of insulin. *Most disposable insulin pens contain 3 mL or 300 units of insulin.*

6. True. Becton Dickinson pen needles are compatible with all insulin pens sold in the United States.

7. True. The expiration date of insulin contained in a cartridge or pen can range from 10-42 days.

8. False. Since needles are removed after each use, it is acceptable to use an insulin pen in more than one person. *Using an insulin pen in more than one person increases the potential risk of transmitting bloodborne pathogens, substances that can cause disease. Therefore, insulin pens should not be shared between persons.*

9. False. Federal regulations determine the disposal of used needles in home settings. *Regulations for home sharps disposal vary by state.*

10. False. Hypotension (high blood pressure) is a major risk factor for heart disease, stroke, congestive heart failure, and kidney disease. *Hypertension (high blood pressure) is a major risk factor for heart disease, stroke, congestive heart failure, and kidney disease.*

11. True. A 10% decrease in total blood cholesterol levels can reduce the incidence of heart disease by as much as 30%.

Fill in the Blank Key

1. Test strip
2. Lancet
3. Insulin
4. Subcutaneously
5. Control
6. Pedometer
7. Hemoglobin A1c
8. 6 24
9. Ostomy
10. Urostomy

Short Answer Key

1. The steps for monitoring blood glucose are as follows:

   a. Gather materials used for test: meter, test strips, lancets, and alcohol preps.

   b. Wash hands or clean finger/area of skin to be used for test with alcohol prep.

   c. Place test strip in meter or obtain test strip from meter.

   d. Lance (stick) the area of skin to obtain blood sample.

   e. Apply blood sample to test strip.

   f. Record blood glucose reading in log book.

   g. Discard lancet in hard, plastic, puncture-resistant container.

2. The steps of insulin injection using a syringe are as follows:

   a. Wash hands; gather materials (insulin vial, syringe, alcohol prep).

   b. Clean site of injection with alcohol prep.

   c. Remove needle cover; draw air into syringe that is equivalent to number of insulin units.

   d. Inject air into insulin vial.

   e. Invert insulin vial, withdraw insulin units, and check for air bubbles while syringe needle remains in vial.

   f. If air bubbles are present, push insulin back into vial and withdraw insulin units again. Repeat until there are no large air bubbles present in syringe.

   g. Remove syringe from vial.

   h. Pinch fold of skin, inject at 45- or 90-degree angle.

   i. Keep needle in skin for a few seconds; then release skin fold and remove needle from skin.

3. The steps for monitoring blood pressure include the following: Avoid food, caffeine, tobacco, and alcohol for 30 minutes before taking a measurement. Eating, drinking caffeine or alcohol, or using tobacco can increase blood pressure readings. Empty your bladder before measuring blood pressure; a full bladder can increase blood pressure slightly. Sit quietly for 3–5 minutes in a comfortable position, with your legs and ankles uncrossed and your back supported against a chair, before measuring blood pressure. Rest your arm, raised to the level of your heart, on a table, desk, or chair arm. You may need to place a pillow or cushion under your arm to elevate it enough. Place the cuff on bare skin, not over clothing. Rolling up a sleeve until it tightens around your arm can result in an inaccurate reading, so you may need to slip your arm out of the sleeve. Place the arm cuff over the brachial artery. There is usually a guide on the cuff for appropriate placement. Make sure to use a cuff that is the correct size for your arm. If a cuff is too small, the blood pressure reading can be falsely elevated. If the cuff is too large, the blood pressure can be lower than the actual measurement. Measure blood pressure by following the directions for the specific monitor. Remain quiet (i.e., don't talk) while taking your blood pressure. If your monitor doesn't automatically log blood pressure readings or heart rates, write the measurements down in your own log. Take a repeat reading 2–3 minutes after the first one to check accuracy. You can wait as little as one minute between readings.

4. A pedometer is a device that records each step a person takes by detecting the motion of the hips. The distance of each person's step varies, so calibration is needed to record a standardized distance, such as the number of miles walked. The recommended number of steps per day for weight loss is 10,000. The use of a pedometer is associated with significant increases in physical activity and significant decreases in body mass index and blood pressure. Pedometer technology includes a mechanical sensor and software to count steps. Early forms of the device used a mechanical switch to detect steps, together with a simple counter. More advanced pedometers rely on microelectromechanical system (MEMS) inertial sensors and sophisticated software to detect steps. The use of MEMS inertial sensors permits more accurate detection of steps and fewer false-positives. A false-positive occurs when the pedometer incorrectly records a step when the device is bumped or moved. The pedometer should be worn on a belt to provide an accurate measurement of steps. The simplest pedometers only count steps and display the number of steps and/or distance. However, there are pedometers that also provide calorie estimates, clocks, timers, stopwatches, speed estimators, and 7-day memory, as well as monitor heart rate.

5. False-negative results can occur if home pregnancy tests are done very early in the pregnancy. False-positive results can be caused by having soap in the urine collection cup, testing equipment in a very warm environment, protein or blood in the urine, or the hCG hormone in the urine from another cause.

Word Search Key

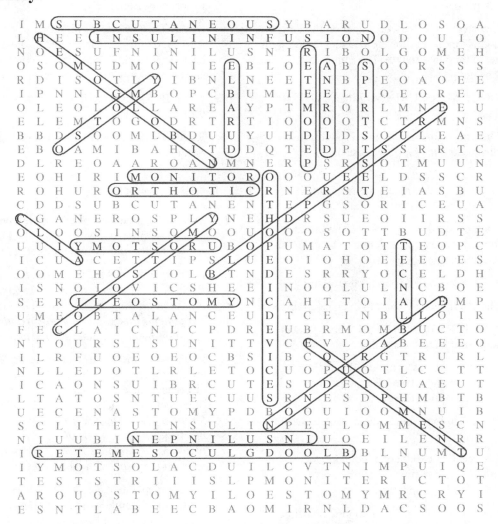

Chapter 19 Answer Keys

Multiple Choice Key

1. b. Specific drug manufacturer or labeler of the product.

2. c. Physicians, pharmacists, nurses, and administrators.

3. d. All of the above.

4. d. All of the above.

5. d. All of the above.

6. c. Similar drug names, package sizes, label format.

7. d. All of the above.

8. a. Expired.

9. d. All of the above.

10. a. Are more efficient and effective in ensuring timely consumer protection than an FDA-initiated court action or seizure of the product.

Matching Key

1. B. II. PRODUCT M.V.I. ADULT (Multi-Vitamin Infusion), 10 mL UNIT VIAL

   REASON: Subpotent (Multiple Ingredient Drug): The discolored top chamber solution does not meet the visual appearance specification. This discoloration potentially impacts the potency of the Biotin and Folic Acid contained in the top chamber.

2. C. III. PRODUCT Fentanyl Transdermal System 75 mcg/hr, 5 systems per box

   REASON: Incorrect NDC bar code label on the outer carton; bar code is indicated for the 100 mcg/hr strength instead of the 75 mcg/hr strength. The immediate package label is correct.

3. C. III. PRODUCT ALLOPURINOL Tablets, USP, 100 mg, 30 Tablets

   REASON: Labeling: Correct Labeled Product Mispack; 100 mg bottles packed in shipping boxes labeled as 300 mg.

4. B. II. PRODUCT Propofol Injectable Emulsion 1%, 200 mg/20 mL, (10 mg/mL), 20 ml vials

   REASON: Lack of Sterility Assurance: The product was manufactured on equipment found to be contaminated with microbiological organisms.

5. A. I. PRODUCT Isosorbide Mononitrate, 60 mg

   REASON: The products may contain oversized tablets.

6. A. I. PRODUCT NIKKI HASKELL'S StarCaps Diet System Dietary Supplement Capsules

   REASON: Unapproved new drug; the dietary supplement lots contain the undeclared drug ingredient Bumetanide, a prescription diuretic.

7. B. II. PRODUCT Liothyronine Sodium Tablets, USP 5 mcg

   REASON: The recall is being conducted due to a stability failure at the 12-month time point; the assay value of this lot was found to be subpotent.

8. B. II. PRODUCT IBUDONE (hydrocodone bitartrate and ibuprofen tablets), 5 mg/200 mg

   REASON: Subpotent (Multiple Ingredient Drug): Below specification for the assay at the room temperature 3-month stability time-point for Ibuprofen and Hydrocodone Bitartrate.

9. C. III. PRODUCT 1) Honey Lemon Soothing Cough Drops (Menthol) 9.1 mg, individually twist wrapped drops

   REASON: Subpotent (Single Ingredient Drug): Cough drops are out of specification for menthol.

10. A. I. PRODUCT Ondansetron in 5% Dextrose Injection, 32 mg/50 mL (0.64 mg/mL), Single-Dose Premix Bag

    REASON: Non-Sterility: This product is being recalled because a white feathery substance found floating inside the IV bag was identified as mold.

11. A. I. RIPPED TABS TR tablets, Anabolic Amplifier Proprietary Blend

    REASON: Marketed without an Approved NDA/ANDA: 62 products marketed as dietary supplements have been found to contain steroid or steroid-like substances, making them unapproved new drugs.

12. C. III. PRODUCT Sertraline Tablets, 50 mg bottles of 90

    REASON: Incorrect medication guides shipped with product.

True or False Key

1. True. A hospital formulary is developed and maintained by a committee of medical and allied health staff called the Pharmacy and Therapeutics (P&T) Committee.

2. False. Formularies are not a concern in retail pharmacy. *Because PBMs and insurance companies use formularies, retail pharmacies need to understand them and assist patients and physicians to maximize savings while maintaining high standards of health care.*

3. False. When there is a request for use of products that are not on the official hospital formulary, the pharmacist must refuse the request and offer a comparable or therapeutically equivalent product. *The pharmacy's nonformulary procedure may or may not restrict the use of various dosage forms of a given chemical entity, so pharmacy technicians need to understand the policy in place at their specific institutions.*

4. False. Independent community pharmacies typically do not become members of a GPO. *Hospitals, independent community pharmacies, and other retail chain pharmacies typically become members of a GPO to leverage buying power and take advantage of the lower prices that manufacturers offer to the GPOs.*

5. True. Purchasing contracts can involve sole-source or multisource products. Sole-source branded products are available from only one manufacturer, whereas multisource generic products are available from numerous manufacturers.

6. False. A GPO guarantees the price of pharmaceuticals over the established contract period, which is usually 3-6 months. *A GPO guarantees the price of pharmaceuticals over the established contract period, which may be 1 year or more.*

7. True. It is important that the pharmacy technician documents any off-contract purchases resulting from manufacturers' inability to supply a given product that

the pharmacy is buying on contract, which may require the pharmacy to buy or substitute a competing product that is not on contract at a higher cost.

8. False. For most pharmacies, the advantages of direct ordering outweigh the disadvantages. *For most pharmacies, the disadvantages of direct ordering outweigh the advantages.*

9. True. Some drugs can only be purchased directly from the manufacturers.

10. False. Borrowing or lending drugs between pharmacies is not allowed due to federal restrictions. *Borrowing or lending drugs between pharmacies is usually restricted to emergency situations and limited to authorized staff.*

11. False. In a reliable and efficient receiving system, the personnel responsible for ordering should be the same as the receiving personnel. *Some pharmacies create processes whereby the person receiving pharmaceuticals is different from the person ordering them. This process is especially important for controlled substances, because it effectively establishes a check in the system to minimize potential drug diversion opportunities.*

12. True. Just as checking the product label carefully is important when a prescription or medication order is filled, taking the same care when receiving pharmaceuticals and accurately placing them in their storage location are essential for prevention of medication errors.

13. False. Research on tall man lettering has failed to demonstrate effectiveness in distinguishing similarities and preventing look-alike, sound-alike drug mix-ups. *Research on tall man lettering has demonstrated effectiveness in distinguishing similarities and preventing look-alike, sound-alike drug mix-ups.*

14. False. If a hospital uses a BCMA system, it is critical that each bar code on items new to the facility be scanned at the time that each product is received to ensure that the product bar code is in the BCMA system. This does not apply to products that have been received before from the same manufacturer. *All items should be scanned, both new and regular. This applies even if the product has been received before from the same manufacturer. Some bar codes contain lot and expiration date information, which could change with each manufacturer batch production.*

15. False. Schedule III, IV, and V controlled substances are generally obtained in a manner identical to that for Schedule II substances. *Schedule III, IV, and V controlled substances are generally obtained in a manner identical to that for non-controlled substances.*

16. True. The difficult logistical and control factors of medication samples have led many organizations to adopt policies that simply disallow medication samples.

Fill in the Blank Key

1. National Drug Code (or NDC number)

2. Formulary

3. Group purchasing organization (GPO)

4. Direct

5. Wholesaler

6. Prime

7. Stock rotation

8. Tall man lettering

9. 6 months

10. Perpetual

11. 222

12. Turns

Short Answer Key

1. In a reliable and efficient receiving system, the receiving personnel verify that the shipment is complete and intact before putting items into circulation or inventory. The receiving process begins with the verification of the boxes containing pharmaceuticals delivered by the shipper. The person receiving the shipment begins the process by verifying that the name and address on the boxes are correct and that the number of boxes matches the shipping manifest. Many drug wholesalers use rigid plastic totes because they protect the contents of each shipment better than foam or cardboard boxes. These totes are also environmentally friendly; they are returned to the wholesaler for cleaning and reuse. Each tote should be inspected for gross damage. Products with a cold storage requirement should be processed first. The shipper is responsible for taking measures to ensure that the cold storage environment is maintained during the shipment process and generally packages these items in a shippable foam cooler that includes frozen cold packs to keep products at the correct storage temperature during shipment.

Receiving personnel play a critical role in protecting the pharmacy from financial responsibility for products damaged in shipment, products not ordered, and products not received. Any obvious damage or other discrepancies with the shipment, such as a breach in the cold storage environment or an incorrect product, should be noted on the shipping manifest; if warranted, that part of the shipment should be refused. Ideally, identifying gross shipment damage or incorrect tote counts should be performed in the presence of the delivery person and should be well documented when signing for the order. Other problems identified after delivery personnel have left such as mispicks, product dating, or internally damaged goods must be resolved according to the vendor's policies. Most vendors have specific procedures to follow in reporting and resolving such discrepancies. The technician can also identify packages that are received containing broken tablets, defective seals, etc., so that the wholesaler/shipper can be alerted to weaknesses in the delivery system. Quality issues can often be identified first by the technicians working the receiving area.

The next step of the receiving process entails checking the newly delivered products against the receiving copy of the purchase order. This generally occurs after the delivery person has left. A purchase order, created when the order is placed, is a complete list of the items that were ordered. Some pharmacies may still use a traditional paper purchase order. However, the state-of-the-art practice employs electronic, Web-based technology to place orders with respective wholesale distributors. In this case, the order is transmitted and received in an instant, and the wholesaler's inventory of particular products is available in near real-time. This technology allows for more efficient operations and effective communication between the pharmacy and wholesaler and simplifies order reconciliation and billing processes. The person responsible for checking products into inventory uses the receiving copy of the purchase order that is included in each wholesaler tote to ensure that the products ordered have been received. The name, brand, dosage form, size of the package, concentration or strength, and quantity of product must match the purchase order.

Once the accuracy of the shipment is confirmed, the packing list is generally signed and dated by the person receiving the shipment. At this point, the product's expiration date should be checked to ensure that it meets the department's minimum expiration date requirement. Frequently, departments require that products received have a minimum shelf life of 6 months remaining before they expire.

If a hospital uses a BCMA system, it is critical that each bar code be scanned at the time that each product is received. This ensures that the product bar code is in the BCMA system so that it can scan correctly when it gets to the bedside. This applies even if the product has been received before from the same manufacturer.

Some bar codes contain lot and expiration date information, which could change with each manufacturer batch production. In the event that a bar code does not scan, it is customary for the receiving technician to add the item to the BCMA system manually or to overlay an internal bar code on the product prior to shelving it.

It is noteworthy to mention that, on occasion, the manufacturer/wholesaler may inadvertently ship an excess quantity of an ordered product to the pharmacy. The ethical response is to immediately notify the manufacturer or wholesaler of this situation and arrange for the return of any excess quantity. If a pharmacist or pharmacy technician other than the receiving technician removes a product from a shipment before it has been properly received and cannot locate the receiving copy of the purchase order, a written record of receipt should be created. This is done by listing the product, dosage form, concentration/strength, package size, and quantity on a blank piece of paper or on the supplier's packing slip/invoice and checking off the line item received. In both cases, the name of the person receiving the product should be included, and the document should be given to the receiving technician to avoid confusion and an unnecessary call to the wholesaler or manufacturer.

2. Controlled substances have specific ordering, receiving, storage, dispensing, inventory, record-keeping, return, waste, and disposal requirements established under the law. The Pharmacist's Manual: An Informational Outline of the Controlled Substances Act of 1970 and the ASHP Technical Assistance Bulletin on Institutional Use of Controlled Substances provide detailed information on the specific handling requirements for controlled substances. It is critical for pharmacy technicians to know two principles regarding controlled substances: 1. Ordering and receiving Schedule II controlled substances require special order forms and additional time (1 to 3 days). 2. Controlled substances are inventoried and tracked continuously. This type of inventory method is referred to as a perpetual inventory process, whereby each dose or packaged unit such as a tablet, vial, or milliliter of fluid volume is accounted for at all times. In some pharmacies, pharmacy technicians work with pharmacists to manage inventory and order, dispense, and store controlled substances.

Controlled substances require additional processing when ordering, receiving, dispensing, storing, and inventorying occurs. These procedures are required by Drug Enforcement Administration (DEA) regulations and, in many cases, the State Board of Pharmacy. These regulations create the chain of accountability in the interest of minimizing drug diversion, illicit drug use, and public safety. State and federal regulations vary regarding length of storage requirements for purchase orders, invoices, and dispensing records. It is best to check both sets of regulations and comply with the stricter requirements. Regulations specific to Schedule II controlled substances require DEA form 222 to be completed to initiate procurement of these products. Form 222 is a triplicate, handwritten form, and each copy has a specific intent, as specified by the DEA. On receipt of DEA Schedule II products, the pharmacy must separately file the appropriate copy of form 222, along with the supplier's copy of the invoice and packing slip accompanying each shipment. Alternatively, the pharmacy can be registered with the DEA to place Schedule II orders online through the wholesaler's electronic process. A perpetual inventory of Schedule II products is maintained by the pharmacy, so an exact accounting should be performed whenever a product is added or removed from the inventory.

Schedule III, IV, and V controlled substances are generally obtained in a manner identical to that for other noncontrolled substances. However, the receipt and storage requirements of these products may depend on state regulation or on the specific employer's policy. For example, state regulation may require a pharmacy to file separately the receipts of all controlled substances ordered during a particular year and to maintain them in a readily retrievable manner for inspection. Some pharmacies may require all controlled substances inventories to be shelved separately from other legend drugs, whereas others may store them together.

3. Because of the hazards inherent with human exposure to antineoplastic or chemotherapy products, care and precaution must be exercised in the receipt, handling, and storage of these products. The distributor generally ships antineoplastic drugs separately and apart from other products (e.g., in their own container). Special care should be exercised when opening and unpacking totes containing these products. Although the distributor takes appropriate measures to pack and pad the items properly inside totes, it is still possible for damage to occur. As an additional safety precaution, many pharmacy operations keep the inventory locations of these products completely separate from those of other medications (usually in a dedicated satellite pharmacy, or the area where the antineoplastic drugs are prepared for patient administration). Pharmacy technicians should be familiar with the organization's chemotherapy and hazardous materials spill management protocol. Most hospitals have a "chemotherapy spill kit" on hand to be used in the management and cleanup of an accidental spill.

4. Investigational drugs also require special ordering, inventorying, and handling procedures. Generally, the use of investigational drugs is categorized into two distinct areas: 1) use under a formal protocol approved by the site's institutional review board (IRB), and 2) the compassionate use of investigational drugs for a single patient as may be authorized by the manufacturer and the FDA. Compassionate drug use is legal, although the drug is technically still being scientifically tested by the manufacturer (usually in a late stage of drug development) and will eventually be considered by the FDA for licensure as it shows promising health benefits. In both cases, the physician or primary investigator may be responsible for ordering the product, whereas the pharmacy staff generally handles the inventory management and distribution of the investigational drug once it is received.

Most research protocols require very rigorous investigational drug inventory and dispensing records, including maintaining a perpetual inventory of the product. Maintaining a perpetual inventory is similar to that required for DEA Schedule II drugs; it means that the pharmacy follows procedures to ensure a complete and accurate accounting of the precise quantity on hand for the drug (down to the single unit of measure). Other record-keeping in this context involves evidence of proper cold chain storage—a complete daily log of product refrigeration temperatures and actions that is taken if the storage temperature range deviated from those required by the product. Research Site Monitors (regulatory administrators) invariably ask to see these records during their periodic site visits. Investigational drug products are typically required under protocol to be stored in a secured area of the pharmacy, physically separate and apart from those noninvestigational products, simply as a matter of preventing an inadvertent dispensing error.

Some pharmacies associated with academic institutions that conduct clinical research have organized investigational drug services that are formally managed by a pharmacist who is principally dedicated to pharmaceutical research activities. In these cases, the investigational drug service pharmacist may have been delegated authority to order, dispense, and manage the inventory of investigational drugs in full compliance with the research protocol. Pharmacy technicians often prepare or handle investigational drugs and participate in the perpetual inventory record-keeping system.

5. The intent of the restricted drug distribution system (RDDS) is to ensure that specific drugs identified as high risk are safely procured, prescribed, dispensed, and administered. The FDA, the manufacturer, and the distributor collaborate to establish tighter controls over

designated products. If improperly administered, certain drugs can cause serious adverse effects such as blood disorders, birth defects, or changes in cardiovascular status. For example, the drug thalidomide can cause severe birth defects. If the clinical benefit of using a restricted drug is perceived to outweigh the risks, the pharmacy can obtain it under prescription if proper screening, education, and monitoring requirements are satisfied. Satisfying the requirements necessary to obtain these drugs may be limited to the presence of a specific disease state being treated by a physician who is registered under the RDDS. As a matter of satisfying restricted distribution requirements, the physician may have to attest to patient-specific criteria. This might include a failed treatment response to other medications, contraindications to other therapy, or evidence from laboratory data. In other cases, physicians may need to commit to administering the medication under controlled conditions such as in their office. In most cases, the RDDS requires registration of the prescribing physician, dispensing pharmacy, patient name and other demographic information, a patient agreement form for liability purposes, the specific indication for the medication, its dose and quantity to be dispensed. In some programs, lab results, adherence to a robust patient counseling or outreach protocol, and reimbursement information guaranteeing payment are required. The primary goal of RDDS is safe, effective product use and reduced risk to the patient. Some examples of medications requiring a RDDS include Abarelix (Plenaxis), Alosetron (Lotronex), Ambrisentan (Letairis), Bosentan (Tracleer), Clozapine (Clozaril), Deferasirox (Exjade), Dofetilide (Tikosyn), Getfitinib (Iressa), Isotretinoin (Accutane), Lenalidomide (Revlimid), Mifepristone (Mifeprex), Natalizumab (Tysabri), Sodium Oxybate (Xyrem), and Thalidomide (Thalomid).

Alphabet Soup Key

a. PO: Purchase Order

b. GPO: Group Purchasing Organization

c. FDA: Food and Drug Administration

d. NDC: National Drug Code

e. DRLS: Drug Registration and Listing System

f. AWP: Average Wholesale Price

g. PBM: Pharmacy Benefits Manager

h. BCMA: Bar Code Medication Administration

i. DEA: Drug Enforcement Administration

j. IRB: Institutional Review Board

k. RDDS: Restricted Drug Distribution System

l. MSDS: Materials Safety Data Sheet

m. DOT: Department of Transportation

n. RCRA: Resource Conservation and Recovery Act

o. EPA: Environmental Protection Agency

p. GMP: Good Manufacturing Practices

q. NDA: New Drug Application

r. ANDA: Abbreviated New Drug Application

s. IMPACT: International Medicinal Products Anti-Counterfeiting Taskforce

t. WHO: World Health Organization

Chapter 20 Answer Keys

Multiple Choice Key

1. d. All of the above.

2. e. All of the above.

3. b. Retrospective.

4. d. All of the above.

5. a. Develop formularies and negotiate discounts or rebates with pharmaceutical companies.

6. d. All of the above.

7. d. All of the above.

8. d. All of the above.

9. a. Pre-paid through payroll taxes.

10. d. Must pay all costs for prescriptions.

Matching Key

1. Part D. Prescription drug coverage

2. Part A. Hospital insurance

3. Part B. Medical insurance

4. Part C. Medicare Advantage plans

5. 7. Brand-Name Drug Mandated by Law: substitution not allowed

6. 5. Brand Name Dispensed at Generic Price: substitution allowed

7. 6. Override

8. 4. Generic not in stock: substitution allowed

9. 2. Patient DAW: substitution allowed; patient requested product dispensed

10. 1. Physician DAW: substitution not allowed by provider

11. 0. Generic or Single-Source Brand: no product selection

12. 9. Other

13. 3. Pharmacist-Selected Brand Name: substitution allowed; pharmacist-selected product

14. 8. Generic not available: substitution allowed

True or False Key

1. False. Typically, the reimbursement formula for a generic product is the same as that for a brand product. *Typically, the reimbursement formula for a generic product is different than that for a brand product.*

2. True. Some third-party payers may pay a higher dispensing fee for generic drugs or formulary products as an incentive to encourage utilization of preferred products.

3. False. In the IPAP model, pharmacies typically receive payment for medications that have already been dispensed. *In the IPAP model, pharmacies typically receive "replacement" product for medications that have already been dispensed.*

4. False. Medicare Part B, which covers outpatient physician and hospital services, clinical laboratory services, and durable medical equipment, prosthetics, orthotics, and supplies (DMEPOS), is automatic medical insurance for those 65 and older. *Medicare Part B is optional medical insurance for outpatient physician and hospital services, clinical laboratory services, and durable medical equipment, prosthetics, orthotics, and supplies (DMEPOS).*

5. True. Medicare Part D is a federal prescription drug program that is paid for by the Centers for Medicare and Medicaid Services (CMS) and by individual premiums.

6. True. Since drug formularies for Medicare Part D vary from plan to plan, beneficiaries must be careful when choosing a Medicare prescription drug plan to ensure that their prescription drugs are covered.

7. False. CMS requires that all Medicare prescription drug plans cover at least six drugs in each of the ten therapeutic categories. *CMS requires that all Medicare prescription drug plans cover at least two drugs in each of the six therapeutic categories.*

8. True. If a beneficiary has a prescription for a drug that requires prior authorization from the Part D plan, the prescribing physician needs to obtain prior authorization for the drug before the claim can be paid.

9. False. All Part D claims must contain a National Provider Identifier (NPI) for the prescriber, or may substitute the provider's DEA number. *All Part D claims must contain a National Provider Identifier (NPI) for the prescriber.*

10. False. Medicaid is another term for Medicare. *Medicaid is a medical and long-term care program that is jointly funded by the federal and state governments. Medicaid covers three main groups of low-income Americans: parents and children, the elderly, and the disabled.*

11. True. As of April 1, 2008, all Medicaid prescriptions must be electronically prescribed or written/printed on "tamper resistant" paper.

12. True. By law, Medicaid recipients may not be denied services based on their inability to pay the assigned cost sharing.

Fill in the Blank Key

1. Revenue
2. Prospective
3. Third-party
4. Copayment
5. AWP
6. Patient assistance programs (PAPs)
7. Pharmacy benefit managers (PBMs)
8. Formulary
9. Diagnosis-related group (DRG)
10. Dual eligible

Short Answer Key

1. Step therapy requires use of a recognized first-line drug before a more complex or expensive second-line drug is used. Beneficiaries must try and fail with the first-line drug before a second-line drug can be covered by the benefit. For example, the PBM might require use of a generic antibiotic before newer, more complex, broad-spectrum antibiotics are prescribed.

2. Patients with a prescription drug benefit should have a prescription identification (ID) card. The information on the prescription ID card is necessary in order to submit

a claim to the PBM. The card identifies the PBM or drug benefit provider. It shows a telephone number for the PBM customer service department. The employer may be identified (Your Company, Inc.), followed by the Member Name (Jane Doe) and Member ID Number (12345678). If the beneficiary is different from the plan member, such as a dependent child, the Participant's Name may be listed. Finally, the BIN # (000012) is the bank identification number, which is also needed to submit the claim. It references the claims processor or PBM. Once the technician enters information in the pharmacy computer from the prescription ID card and the prescription, the PBM either accepts or rejects the claim. If the claim is rejected, the PBM responds with a message, commonly known as a rejection code. Such codes are standard across all prescription benefit plans and may include "Missing or Invalid Patient ID," "Prior authorization required," "Pharmacy not contracted with plan on date of service," "Refill too soon," or "Missing or invalid quantity prescribed." The technician must assess the meaning of the rejection code and respond accordingly. The resolution may be simple, such as checking the patient ID and making sure it was entered correctly. Or the pharmacist or physician may need to take further action (e.g., obtaining prior authorization) in order for the claim to be processed. If the issue can't be resolved or if the rejection code is unclear, the technician may need to call the PBM customer service, which is usually listed on the prescription ID card.

3. Prospective payment typically includes all costs associated with treating a particular condition, including medications. With prospective payment systems, pharmacies are challenged to deliver drugs at or below the predetermined rate in order to ensure that drug costs are covered. More information on prospective payment methods is presented later in this chapter. In community pharmacy practice, the most common type of payment method is retrospective or fee for service. In the retrospective payment model, drugs are dispensed, and later reimbursed, according to a predetermined formula that is specified in a contract between the pharmacy and the third-party payer, such as the insurance company or pharmacy benefit manager.

4. Many drug companies offer certain free drugs through patient assistance programs (PAPs) to low-income patients who lack prescription drug coverage and meet certain criteria. The criteria for PAPs are widely variable and are determined by individual drug companies. In most cases, the products that are available free to the patient are proprietary drugs, and the patient is required to complete an application that determines eligibility. On approval, the drug company delivers a specified quantity of the drug (usually a 30- to 90-day supply) to a licensed pharmacist or physician on the patient's behalf. Some companies also offer bulk replacement or institutional patient assistance programs (IPAPs). In the IPAP model, medications are provided to an institution (e.g., pharmacy or clinic) rather than to the individual patient. The institution has the obligation of verifying that each patient who receives medications meets the established criteria. In the IPAP model, pharmacies typically receive "replacement" product for medications that have already been dispensed. Pharmacy technicians can play an important role in helping pharmacists identify and enroll eligible patients in Patient Assistance Programs. RX for Success Copay foundations or independent charity patient assistance programs are other resources that can be used to help patients who can't afford to pay for prescriptions or copays.

Crossword Puzzle Key

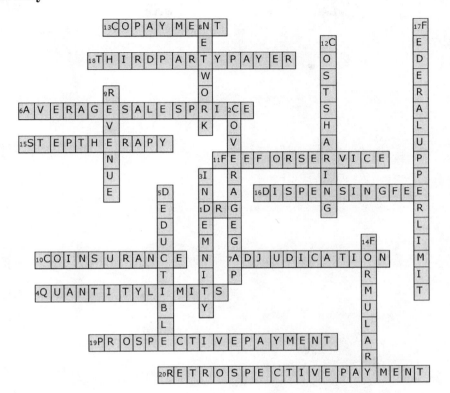

Index

A

absorption factors, 63

accrediting agencies, 19

adverse effects, 55

alphabet soup, community and ambulatory care
practice, 16, 131

    drug classifications, 62, 157

    drug information resources, 39, 146

    hospital practice, 22, 135

    inventory control, 113, 190

    law, 11, 127-128

    medication dosage, 72, 164

    pharmacologic actions, 62, 157

    processing orders, prescriptions, 78, 167-
168

    purchasing, 113, 190

    routes of administration, 72, 164

ambulatory care practice, learning outcomes, 13

ambulatory pharmacy, 1

aseptic technique, learning outcomes, 91

B

background information, 35

billing, learning outcomes, 115

biopharmaceutics, 63

blood glucose meters, 103

blood pressure monitors, 103

buccal administration, 69

C

capsules, 69

centralized pharmacy, 19

certification, 1

communications, learning outcomes, 41

community pharmacy practice, learning outcomes,
13

compounding, 85

    equipment, 85

contamination, 91

continuous glucose monitoring systems, 103

continuous infusion pumps, 103

controlled substances, 7

crossword puzzle

    aseptic technique, 95, 178

    billing, 119, 192

    community and ambulatory care practice,
17, 132

    home care, 29, 138

    human body, 53, 153

    IV admixtures, 95, 178

    medication dosage, 73, 164

    pharmacy, 5, 125

    pharmacy calculations, 83, 170

    reimbursement, 119, 192

    routes of administration, 73, 164

    sterile compounding, 95, 178

cytotoxic drug handling, 91

D

decentralized pharmacy, 19
decimals, 79
disease states, 63
diseases, 47
disorders, 47
drug
    classifications, learning outcomes, 55
    distribution methods, 19
    information request, 35
    information resources, learning outcomes, 35
    interactions, 63
    names, 55
    therapy, 47
durable medical equipment, 103

E

elimination, 63
emulsions, 69
ephedrine, 7
expiration dates, 25

F

FDA approval process, 7
fill in the blank
    aseptic technique, 94, 175-176
    billing, 118, 191
    communication and teamwork, 44, 148-149
    community and ambulatory care practice, 16, 130
    drug classifications, 60-61, 156
    drug information resources, 38, 144
    home care, 28, 136-137
    hospital practice, 22, 134
    human body, 51-52, 152
    inventory control, 113, 187
    IV admixtures, 94, 175-176
    law, 10, 127
    medical equipment, devices, supplies, 106, 183
    medication dosage, 72, 161
    medication errors, 100, 179
    nonsterile compounding, repackaging, 89, 172
    pharmaceutics, pharmacodynamics, pharmacokinetics, 66, 158
    pharmacologic actions, 60-61, 156
    pharmacy, 4, 123
    pharmacy calculations, 82, 169
    processing orders, prescriptions, 78, 166
    purchasing, 113, 187
    reimbursement, 118, 191
    routes of administration, 72, 161
    specialty practice, 34, 140
    sterile compounding, 94, 175-176
formal training, 1
formulary system, 109
fractions, 79

G

generic drug substitution, 7
granules, 69

H

hazardous drug handling, 91
heart rate monitors, 103
high alert medications, 97
home care
    diseases, conditions, 25
    goals, 25
    learning outcomes, 25
    team, 25
home diagnostic products, 103
home infusion therapy, 25
hospital practice, learning outcomes, 19
human body structure, function, learning objectives, 47

I

infusion systems, 25

institutional pharmacy, 1

insulin

    delivery, 103

    pens, 103

Internet research

    drug information resources, 39, 146-147

    pharmacy, 4, 124

    specialty practice, 34, 142

intravenous drug therapy, 91

inventory control, learning outcomes, 109

IV admixtures, learning outcomes, 91

L

lab monitoring, 103

labeling, 109

laminar airflow workbench, 91

law, learning outcomes, 7

licensing, 1

liquid medications, 69

lozenges, 69

M

matching

    aseptic technique, 93, 174-175

    billing, 117, 190-191

    communication and teamwork, 43, 148

    community and ambulatory care practice, 14-15, 129

    drug classifications, 58, 154

    drug information resources, 37, 143

    home care, 27, 136

    hospital practice, 20-21, 133

    human body, 49-50, 151

    inventory control, 111-112, 185-186

    IV admixtures, 93, 174-175

    law, 9, 126

    medical equipment, devices, supplies, 105, 182-183

    medication dosage, 71, 160-161

    medication errors, 99, 178-179

    nonsterile compounding, repackaging, 87-

    88, 170-171

    pharmaceutics, pharmacodynamics, pharmacokinetics, 65, 157-158

    pharmacologic actions, 58, 154

    pharmacy, 3, 122

    pharmacy calculations, 81, 168

    processing orders, prescriptions, 77, 165

    purchasing, 111-112, 185-186

    reimbursement, 117, 190-191

    routes of administration, 71, 160-161

    specialty practice, 33, 139

    sterile compounding, 93, 174-175

measurement conversions, 79

medical devices, equipment, learning outcomes, 103

medication

    distribution, 63

    label, 75

    management, 19

    order components, 75

    therapy management, 1

medication dosages, 69, 160

    learning outcomes, 69, 160

medication errors, learning outcomes, 97

multiple choice

    aseptic technique, 92, 174

    billing, 116, 190

    communication and teamwork, 42, 148

    community and ambulatory care practice, 14, 129

    drug classifications, 56-58, 153-154

    drug information resources, 36-37, 142-143

    home care, 26, 136

    hospital practice, 20, 133

    human body, 48-49, 150-151

    inventory control, 110-111, 185

    IV admixtures, 92, 174

    law, 7, 126

    medical equipment, devices, supplies, 104, 182

    medication dosage, 70, 160

    medication errors, 98-99, 178

    nonsterile compounding, repackaging, 86, 170

    pharmaceutics, pharmacodynamics,

pharmacokinetics, 64, 157
pharmacologic actions, 56-58, 153-154
pharmacy, 2, 122
pharmacy calculations, 80, 168
processing orders, prescriptions, 76, 165
purchasing, 110-111, 185
reimbursement, 116, 190
routes of administration, 70, 160
specialty practice, 32, 139
sterile compounding, 92, 174-175

N

nondurable medical equipment, 103
nonsterile compounding, repackaging, learning
    outcomes, 85
nonverbal communications, 41
nuclear medicine, 31
nuclear practice, 31

O

orthopedic support products, 103
ostomy products, 103
outpatient services, 1

P

packaging, 109
parenteral administration, 69
patient
        communication, 13
        privacy, 7
        profile, 75
        safety, 19
pedometers, 103
percentages, 79
pharmaceutical care, 1
pharmaceutical disposal, 109
pharmaceutical receiving, storing, 109
pharmaceutics, learning outcomes, 63
pharmacists, 1
pharmacodynamics, learning outcomes, 63
pharmacokinetics, learning outcomes, 63

pharmacologic actions, learning outcomes, 55
pharmacy
        calculations, learning outcomes, 79
        learning outcomes, 1
        practice, 7
pharmacy technician, 1
        community and ambulatory care practice,
        13
        medication management and, 19
        nuclear practice, 31
        patient communication, 13
policy and procedure manuals, 19
powders, 69
practice sites, 13
prescription
        components, 75
        drug inserts, 7
        filling, 13
pricing benchmarks, 115
processing orders, prescriptions, learning
    outcomes, 75
product formulation, 63
pseudoephedrine, 7
purchasing, learning outcomes, 109

Q

quality assurance monitoring, 97
quality control, 19
quality improvement, 19

R

radioactivity, 31
recalls, 109
record keeping, 85
registration, 1
regulatory agencies, 19
reimbursement, learning outcomes, 115
repackaging medications, 85
routes of administration, learning outcomes, 69,
    160

short answer
  aseptic technique, 94, 176-177
  billing, 118, 191-192
  communication and teamwork, 44, 149
  community and ambulatory care practice, 16, 130-131
  drug classifications, 61, 156
  drug information resources, 39, 144-146
  home care, 28, 137-138
  hospital practice, 22, 134
  human body, 52, 152
  inventory control, 113, 187-190
  IV admixtures, 94, 176-177
  law, 11, 127
  medical equipment, devices, supplies, 106, 184
  medication dosage, 72, 162-163
  medication errors, 100, 180-181
  nonsterile compounding, repackaging, 89, 172-173
  pharmaceutics, pharmacodynamics, pharmacokinetics, 66, 159
  pharmacologic actions, 61, 156
  pharmacy, 4, 123-124
  pharmacy calculations, 82, 169
  processing orders, prescriptions, 78, 166-167
  purchasing, 113, 187-190
  reimbursement, 118, 191-192
  routes of administration, 72, 162-163
  specialty practice, 34, 140-142
  sterile compounding, 94, 176-177
solutions, 69
special handling, 109
special patient populations, 41
special precautions, 55
specialty practice, learning outcomes, 31
state laws, regulations, 7
state prescription monitoring programs, 7
sterile compounding, learning outcomes, 91
sterile products labeling, 25
storage, 109
sublingual administration, 69
supplies, learning outcomes, 103

suspensions, 69
syringes, 103

T
tablets, 69
teamwork, learning outcomes, 41
technology, 19
third-party payers, 19
  billing procedures, 115
  claim, 115
total parenteral nutrition solution, 91
true or false
  aseptic technique, 93, 175
  billing, 118, 191
  communication and teamwork, 43, 148
  community and ambulatory care practice, 15, 129
  drug classifications, 59-60, 154-156
  drug information resources, 38, 143-144
  home care, 27, 136
  hospital practice, 21, 133
  human body, 50-51, 151-152
  inventory control, 112, 186-187
  IV admixtures, 93, 175
  law, 10, 126
  medical equipment, devices, supplies, 106, 183
  medication dosage, 71-72, 161
  medication errors, 99-100, 179
  nonsterile compounding, repackaging, 88, 171-172
  pharmaceutics, pharmacodynamics, pharmacokinetics, 66, 158
  pharmacologic actions, 59-60, 154-156
  pharmacy, 3, 122-123
  pharmacy calculations, 82, 168-169
  processing orders, prescriptions, 77-78, 165-166
  purchasing, 112, 186-187
  reimbursement, 118, 191
  routes of administration, 71-72, 161
  specialty practice, 33, 140
  sterile compounding, 93, 175

U
USP 797, 91

V
verbal communications, 41
veterinary practice compounding, 31

W
word search
    communication and teamwork, 45, 150
    community and ambulatory care practice, 17, 132
    home care, 30, 139
    hospital practice, 23, 135
    law, 12, 128
    medical equipment, devices, supplies, 107, 185
    medication errors, 101, 182
    nonsterile compounding, repackaging, 90, 174
    pharmaceutics, pharmacodynamics, pharmacokinetics, 67, 160
    pharmacy, 6, 125
working relationships, 41

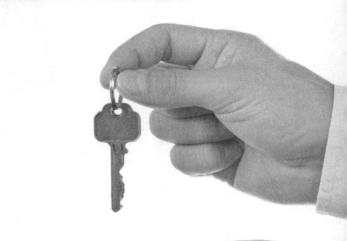
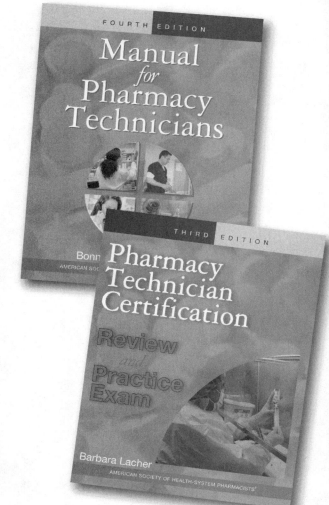
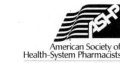
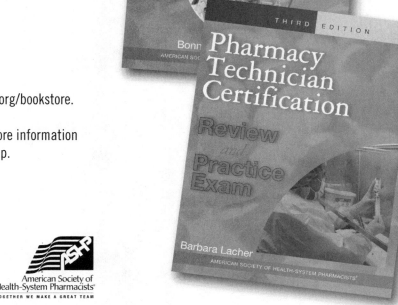

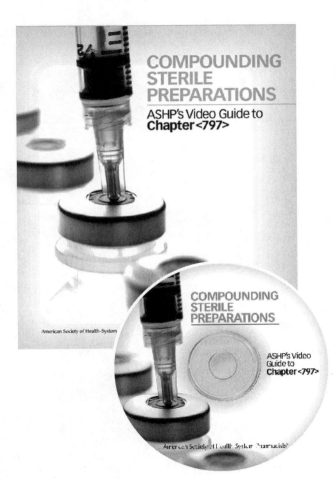
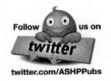
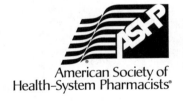

Notes

Notes

Notes

Notes

Notes

Notes